THE NAVAJO SOUND SYSTEM

Studies in Natural Language and Linguistic Theory

VOLUME 55

The titles published in this series are listed at the end of this volume.

THE NAVAJO SOUND SYSTEM

by

JOYCE MCDONOUGH

University of Rochester,
Department of Linguistics,
Rochester NY, U.S.A.

KLUWER ACADEMIC PUBLISHERS
DORDRECHT / BOSTON / LONDON

A C.I.P. Catalogue record for this book is available from the Library of Congress.

ISBN 1-4020-1351-5 (HB)
ISBN 1-4020-1352-3 (PB)

Published by Kluwer Academic Publishers,
P.O. Box 17, 3300 AA Dordrecht, The Netherlands.

Sold and distributed in North, Central and South America
by Kluwer Academic Publishers,
101 Philip Drive, Norwell, MA 02061, U.S.A.

In all other countries, sold and distributed
by Kluwer Academic Publishers,
P.O. Box 322, 3300 AH Dordrecht, The Netherlands.

Printed on acid-free paper

Printed in the Netherlands.

To

Mary McDonough
(1914 - 2002)

And

Kenneth L. Hale
(1934 - 2001)

Each, in vivid memory

TABLE OF CONTENTS

PREFACE

The Navajo language is spoken by the Navajo people who live in the Navajo Nation, located in Arizona and New Mexico in the southwestern United States. The Navajo language belongs to the Southern, or Apachean, branch of the Athabaskan language family. Athabaskan languages are closely related by their shared morphological structure; these languages have a productive and extensive inflectional morphology. The Northern Athabaskan languages are primarily spoken by people indigenous to the sub-artic stretches of North America. Related Apachean languages are the Athabaskan languages of the Southwest: Chiricahua, Jicarilla, White Mountain and Mescalero Apache.

While many other languages, like English, have benefited from decades of research on their sound and speech systems, instrumental analyses of indigenous languages are relatively rare. There is a great deal of work to do before a chapter on the acoustics of Navajo comparable to the standard acoustic description of English can be produced. The kind of detailed phonetic description required, for instance, to synthesize natural sounding speech, or to provide a background for clinical studies in a language is well beyond the scope of a single study, but it is necessary to begin this greater work with a fundamental description of the sounds and supra-segmental structure of the language. In keeping with this, the goal of this project is to provide a baseline description of the phonetic structure of Navajo, as it is spoken on the Navajo reservation today, to provide a foundation for further work on the language.

This project was made feasible by the availability of an extraordinary documentation done over the past 60 years by Robert Young and William Morgan. This year is the 60th anniversary of the publication of the first Young and Morgan grammar. Their principle output (Young and Morgan 1943, 1980, 1987, 1992 and Young 2002) forms the primary reference grammars and dictionaries for Navajo. This body of work makes the Navajo language the most thoroughly documented indigenous language in this hemisphere, and arguably the best documented indigenous language in the world. The Young and Morgan dictionary is word-based, because, as Robert Young has said, that's the way the Navajo wanted it. The Athabaskan languages are primarily verbal, the morphology is highly productive and the inflection is prefixal. The dictionary entries are fully inflected forms. To accomplish this, Young and Morgan worked out the essential paradigms in Navajo and a system of combining and cross-listing them, so that for any given verb word it is possible to conjugate it in any of the aspectual forms it can appear in, and to take the paradigmatic forms and analyze their morphemes, which are also individually cross-referenced. Every entry is accompanied by examples of the word's use in a larger utterance; the examples were collected, not constructed.The documentation of the paradigms alone is a major intellectual accomplishment; since Navajo is an oral culture, they were not working from texts. *The Navajo Language* is, in effect, a fully realized theory of the lexicon for one type of language with a highly productive morphology, combined with extensive documentation of the language's use. The grammar is notoriously hard to casually pick up and use, but that is a statement of our unfamiliarity with the structure of the language, not a statement about the structure of the grammar.

Young and Morgan's 1980 and 1987 *The Navajo Language,* together with the 1992 *Analytic Lexicon* and Young 2000's overview of the verb, *The Navajo Verb System,* are the primary reference resources on Navajo. Notwithstanding the impressive breadth of the Young and Morgan work, the grammars only briefly address the phonetics of the language's sound system. This monograph on the phonetics of the Navajo sound system is intended as a companion to the Young and Morgan grammars. It is meant to provide a baseline description of the sound system and the phonetic details of the consonant and vowels of Navajo. The study is based on the grammars and on an instrumental analysis of recordings collected from speakers who live in the Navajo Nation today.

The study is based on several sets of recordings made over the last nine years. In these recordings, Navajo speakers were asked to recite words from specially prepared wordlists that were constructed to exemplify particular aspects of the sound contrasts, morphological structure and prosody of Navajo. The recordings used in this monograph are grouped into three main data sets: the first made in 1992, a second set in 1995, and a third set in January 2001. The 1992 and 2001 data sets were made at Diné College in Shiprock, New Mexico. This work was funded by the NIH/NIDCD and NSF respectively. The earlier recordings were made at Diné College (then Navajo Community College) in association with Peter Ladefoged and Helen George of UCLA and Clay Slate of NCC. The 1995 data set includes a set of recordings of monolingual speakers made at Navajo Mountain on the reservation, funded by a grant from the American Philosophical Society. This fieldwork was accomplished under the direction of Martha Austin-Garrison. The 2001 data collection was accomplished under the direction of Ms. Austin-Garrison and Anthony Goldtooth Sr. of Diné College. Ms Austin-Garrison was present at all the recording sessions reported on in this monograph, and was a principal in the construction of all the word lists used in the study.

Other consultants were Dr. Mary Willie, University of Arizona, and Anthony Goldtooth Sr., Diné College. I benefited from conversations with Ellavina Perkins, Lorene Legah, Roseann Willinik, Helen George, Linda Platero, Paul Platero and the members of the Language Acquisition class at the Navajo Language Academy (NLA), July 1999 in Rehoboth, New Mexico. I would also like to extend my thanks to Dr. Peggy Speas and the Board of Directors of NLA for providing the opportunity to teach at the summer academy. My gratitude also to Robert Young, Ken Hale, Eloise Jelinek, Doug Whalen, Ian Maddieson, Caroline Smith, Sharon Hargus, Ted Fernald, Carlotta Smith, Sally Rice, Marianne Mithun, Karen Michelson, and Abby Cohn for their support, ideas and help. I thank Bob Ladd for the opportunity to give a seminar on this material at the University of Edinburgh in May 2001. Peter Ladefoged started me on this project, while I was a postdoc under him at UCLA, and though he's not responsible for any errors in these pages, he's been a guiding presence. I'm grateful to my colleagues at the University of Rochester: Greg Carlson, Katherine Crosswhite, Jeff Runner, Rachel Sussman, Ida Toivonen, Mike Tanenhaus, and the members of the U of R Language Science community. Special mention goes to my editor, Scott Stoness. Also to Mark Barton, Dorothy Caulfield, David and Ann Pears, Michael Singer, Claire Waters, Stephen Watson, and Mary Willie. And, as always, my daughter Emma Griffin.

Two very important people died while I was finishing this book: my godmother, Mary McDonough, and my teacher, Ken Hale. This book is dedicated to them.

The book was supported by a grant from the NSF (SES 99-73765) and by a Bellagio fellowship from the Rockefeller Foundation.

November 2002, Rochester N.Y.

Chapter 1

INTRODUCTION

1.0   THE NAVAJO SOUND SYSTEM

The goal of this study is to provide a baseline description of the sound system of Navajo which can be used as a foundation for further work on the language. There are several reasons why a phonetic description of the sound system is important. First, there is little explicit information available about the phonetic details of Navajo or of any language indigenous to this continent. This kind of information is essential to an adequate account of the phonology and morphology of Navajo, as it is in English or in any language. Without it we are dependent on orthography and on descriptions by linguists who have worked on these languages. While these are valuable descriptions, it is difficult, if not impossible, to reconstruct the habits of a speech community based on these accounts, so they need to be supported by instrumental analyses[1].

Understanding the phonology is necessary to a phonetic description. It is possible to provide a phonological sketch of a sound system without an explicit description of the phonetics, but this undertaking is limited by what cannot be encoded in a writing or transcription system. This is especially true of understudied languages, where we are dependent on smaller bodies of documentation.

In Navajo for example, there is a contrast between two sounds written as *s* and *z* in both the Navajo orthography and the IPA. First, this contrast is contextually determined, and not phonemic as the term is usually understood, and second, despite the orthography, it is probably best accounted for as a fortis-lenition distinction and not a voicing contrast, as in Holton (2002) for Tanacross Athabaskan. As discussed in Chapter 5, the fricatives in Navajo exhibit phonological voicing alternations that vary along more parameters than simply laryngeal activity. They vary in manner of articulation and in degree of voicing, and their variance is determined by the fricative's place of articulation. Thus the phonetic realization of phonological 'voicing' environment is a result of several factors; its place of articulation, the following vowel, the fricative's position in the utterance, its domain affiliation, and, finally, by the lack of a clear distinction between

1

fricatives and approximants in the sound system. The process may be best understood as lenition, which is harder to state phonologically and may or may not be the concern of phonology depending on the theoretical framework that is used. But the phonetic behavior of the fricatives under voicing is not recoverable from the orthography, the IPA symbols or from the descriptions of the segments. The intervocalic position is apparently a position of lenition in Athabaskan; the fricatives tend to become more like the surrounding vowels. The output of the process for a fricative contrast is dependent on general physiology (fricatives in general don't voice easily), and the language specific aspects of the sound system. Without instrumental studies, these details are lost.

Interacting with the phonetics is typology. Navajo is polysynthetic and morphologically complex. The lexicon is primarily verbal; true nouns are simple monosyllabic stems (YM:g1-8) that make up a small part of the lexicon. Morphologically complex languages in general lack a substantial body of documentation, and the type of in-depth analyses that are available for more commonly studied languages do not exist for these languages. The morphological structure of the Navajo verb underlies a major part of the lexicon, and its distributional properties, like its rigid ordering constraints, are likely to affect patterns that emerge from the lexicon. The phonetic profile of the word is inherently tied to its morphology, thus documentation of its phonetic structure is necessarily, and I will argue essentially, tied to the morphological structure.

Finally, several important theoretical notions that underlie contemporary phonological theory, such as phonemic contrast, hierarchical structure, minimal pairs, and phonological alternations, are based on detailed knowledge of a few languages where these patterns interact with each other in well-known ways. It is important to understand how these ideas operate in systems that are structurally different from those on which the knowledge base was built. For instance, defining phonemic contrast as a broadly available vehicle for building functional contrasts in a grammar is one of the most solid principles in contemporary language research. But, as we see demonstrated in Navajo, constraints on the distribution of phonemes in the lexicon can undermine the notion of functional contrast, as it is usually interpreted, and lead us to an understanding of the limits of these notions as tools of analysis.

1.1   THE NAVAJO INVENTORY

The phonemic inventories of the languages of the Athabaskan family are all quite similar. They share a complex consonantal inventory with a similar system of manner and laryngeal contrasts on stops and affricates, they all have coronal heavy systems, and most have consonant harmony systems, though they differ in the number of coronal fricatives they exhibit. Labials are rare. The vowel systems are fairly similar, with length and nasality contrasts; some, like Navajo, also have tone contrasts (Krauss 1964, Krauss and Leer 1976, 1981).

The consonantal phonemes of Navajo can be divided into two main groups: the stops and the fricative series. The stops include the plain stops and the affricates. There are two kinds of affricates, classified according to their release: fricated and laterally released. The fricative group, on the other hand, includes not only the fricatives but also the glides and the nasals for reasons discussed in Chapter 3. In this first section, I give an outline of the consonant inventory as a whole, as a point of reference in the book.

Table 1 Navajo consonants in the orthography of Young and Morgan 1987.

p	t, d, t'			k, g, k'	kw, gw '
	ts, dz, ts'	ch, j, ch'			
	tl, dl, tl'				
	s, z	sh, zh		x, gh	h
	ł, l				
m	n				
w			y		

Table 1 shows the Navajo consonants as given by Young and Morgan (1980, 1987). This is the standard orthography in use by Navajo educators. Navajo words in this orthography will be written in italics in the text. When it is given, an IPA transcription will be provided in square brackets, as such: *yishcha* [jɪʃtʃʰah]. In the text, the IPA transcriptions are phonemic. The phonetic IPA transcriptions will be given only in the context of a discussion of the phonetic properties of a sound (primarily in Chapters 4 and 5). Table 2 represents the Navajo stop phonemes in the IPA transcription.

The consonant phonemes are divided by virtue of their phonemic characteristics into stops and fricatives. The stops series exhibit a three-way laryngeal contrast, aspirated, unaspirated and 'glottalized'. The glottalized consonants are ejectives with, as we will see, a distinct timing profile. The unaspirated stops are not voiced. The stops of Navajo contrast in place of articulation: labial, coronal and velar. Coronal consonants in the lexicon far outnumber the labial and velars, so the place of articulation distinction has less contrastive load in than might appear from the table. The labial consonants *b* and *m* are uncommon segments, appearing in only a handful of morphs. Furthermore the *b*, an unaspirated labial stop, does not have the full set of laryngeal and manner contrasts that the other stops have. Outside of these rare labials, there are only two primary places of articulation in Navajo: coronal and velar. Each of these may be further subdivided into two groups: the coronal affricates and fricatives being either anterior or non-anterior, and the velar stops being either labialized or not, though as noted the labial and labialized consonants are rare.

Table 2 Navajo stops in IPA transcription.

	labial	alveolar	palato-alveolar	velar	labialized velar	glottal
plain	p	tx t t'		kx k k'	kxʷ kʷ	ʔ
affricate		tsʰ ts ts'	tʃʰ tʃ tʃ'			
laterally released		tɬʰ tɬ tɬ'				

In Table 3 are the Navajo fricatives and sonorants in the IPA transcription. The fricatives are have voiced and voiceless reflexes. The *h* symbol represents two different sound depending on its syllable position: in syllable-initial position it represents the voiceless velar fricative, in syllable-final position it represents a glottal fricative. The alveolo-palatal fricatives *sh* and *zh*, the voiced velar fricative *gh* and the affricates *ts, tl* and *ch* are all represented with digraphs. Similar orthographies can be found in Hoijer (1945), Sapir-Hoijer (1967), Hale (1972), Kari (1976) Reichard (1952). The orthography is not strictly phonemic; we will discuss this fact below.

Table 3 Navajo fricatives and sonorants in IPA transcription.

	labial	alveolar	palato-alveolar	palatal	velar	labio-velar	glottal
fricative		s z	ʃ ʒ	ç	x ɣ	ɣʷ	h
nasal	m	n					
approximants	w			j	ɥ		

Differences in the descriptions of the sounds in the literature are found primarily in the place of articulation of velar fricatives, and in the characterization of the glides and approximants. Young and Morgan characterize the fricatives and stops in the *k* series as velars or 'back palatals' (1986:xii). I classify them here using the symbol for velar place of articulation. We will take up this discussion in the sections on the phonetic properties of the segment classes in chapter 4 and 5. The descriptions of the glides vary, depending on different phonological considerations that will be considered in Chapter 3.

The fricative group in Table 3 includes the fricatives, approximants, glides and nasals. This group is distinguished from the stop series by their tendency to show contextual alternations. Most of the sounds in the fricative series have a characteristic phonological pattern; they appear as one of three contextual reflexes: voiced, voiceless, and the so-called 'd-effect' alternation. (The d-effect introduces an initial period of closure to the fricative.) Table 4 shows the reflexes of the fricatives as they appear in the lexicon. Understanding these reflexes is important to cross-referencing the entries in the YM grammar, since stems are listed in their voiced reflex.

Table 4 Fricative Reflexes (in the YM orthography).

Voiceless	s	sh	ł	s	s	h
Voiced	z	zh	l	y	y	y
D-effect	dz	ch	dl	dz	d	g

Note that the reflexes in the voiced context of the last three sounds are glides. While orthographically they are similar, these glides differ in their realization according to their nature. The glide reflex of the *s* is a palatal glide, while the reflex of the *h*, a velar fricative, is an approximant or fricative that is strongly co-articulated with the following vowel. This alternation pattern is discussed in Chapters 3 and 5 (see also McDonough 1990).

In the 'd-effect' alternation, a period of closure is introduced to the consonant when it is in stem-initial position by the adjacency of a *d* segment (Sapir-Hoijer 1967, Howren 1971). The nasals are included in the fricative series and not the stop series by nature of the fact that they also exhibit a d-effect alternation: they appear as glottalized nasals under the d-effect condition (Sapir 1925). It is not intended as a theoretical claim about the representation of nasals as a class. The d-effect is discussed in more detail in Chapter 3.

There are several interesting properties that are characteristic of the Navajo fricative gesture in both the affricates and fricatives. The most striking properties are the strength of the frication; this includes the aspiration period of aspirated stops and the constricted quality of the fricative articulation and the fricative-like quality of the sonorants (excluding nasals). These will be discussed in Chapter 5, on the aspectual characteristics of the sounds.

1.2 VOWELS

There are four Navajo principal vowels qualities in the phonemic inventory, shown below in Figure 1. The Navajo vowel system lacks a high back vowel.

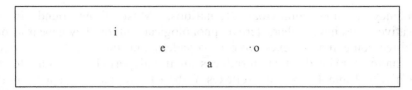

Figure 1 The four principal Navajo vowel qualities.

Navajo vowels contrast in length, tone and nasality. The set of length and nasality contrasts are shown in Figure 2: long and short for both oral and nasal vowels. Furthermore, the high front vowel shows a vowel quality difference between the long and short versions; this is not reflected in the orthography. The standard Athabaskan diacritic for nasality in vowels is a hook beneath the vowel.

short oral		long oral	
i		ii	
e	o	ee	oo
a		aa	
short nasal		long nasal	
į		įį	
ę	ǫ	ęę	ǫǫ
ą		ąą	

Figure 2 Navajo vowel contrasts (excluding tone) in the Navajo orthography.

Both long and short vowels are marked for either high or low tone. In Navajo orthography, high tone is marked with an acute accent, *'á-, 'ą́-, 'áá-,' ą́ą́-,* and low tone unmarked, *'a-, 'ą-, 'aa-,' ąą-.* The default vowel and by far the most common vowel is the short high front *i,* though there is variability in the pronunciation of this vowel depending on context. A full discussion of the vowels, vowel quality distinctions and the vowel space is found in Chapter 5.

1.3 PHONOTACTICS AND PHONEMES

A decisive aspect of the sound system is that the phonemic contrasts that are listed in Table 1 and Figure 2 only occur in stems. The scope of this distribution fact becomes apparent when one looks at the Navajo morphological template in Table 1.2 from Young and Morgan (1980:g107) The stem slot is the rightmost column in the table (labeled STEM in Table 5); it's the rightmost morpheme in the word and a wide range of prefixes may attach to it[2]. The consonantal phonemic contrasts occur only in the onset of the last syllable in the verb; the vocalic contrasts in the nucleus of this syllable.

Table 5 The 'position class' template of Young and Morgan (YM87:g37-38).

0	I					II	III	IV	V	VI			VII	VIII	IX	X
	a	b	c	d	e					a	b	c				STEM

In all the other columns, phonemic contrasts have been severely neutralized. The set of these pre-stem phonemes are listed in (1). The sounds in parentheses appear in only a single morpheme apiece. I have not included sounds (such as *zh, dz*) that occur only as contextual reflexes.

(1)   s, z, sh, d, n, y h, (ł), (l), (j) (b)

The rich inventory in Table 1 is reduced to the unaspirated coronal stop *d*, the coronal fricatives *s, z, sh,* the nasal *n*, the approximant *y,* and the velar fricative *h*. Nearly all manner and place contrasts are neutralized. Inflectional morphemes make up a large set of morphemes in the language; YM (:g302) lists only 550 separate verbal roots, though there are well over 15,000 entries in the dictionary[3]. The set of phonemes used by the inflectional system in this highly inflectional language is not much larger than the set of inflectional phonemes in English. The consonantal inventory in Table 1 is a list of the possible stem onsets, and the vocalic inventory a list of the stem vowels.

Because of this restrictive phonemic distribution, the concept of a phonemic inventory is somewhat misleading as it is usually interpreted; the contrasts are limited to a single position within a multi-syllabic word. An investigation of the phonetic properties of the consonantal phonemic inventory is a study of the onsets of stems. To get a true picture of the sound system, as reflective of the speech habits of the Navajo speaking community, a broader investigation is needed. The distributional asymmetries are likely to be determing factors in the definition of the prosody and in the lexicon, for instance. One thing is clear: the phoneme distribution is determined by the morphological structure of the Navajo language. As the vocabulary of the Athabaskan languages is primarily

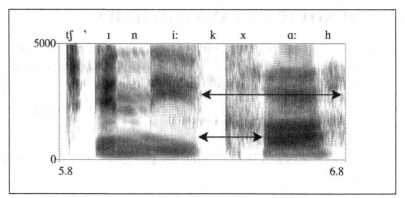

Figure 3 Spectrogram of *ch'íniikaah* [tʃ'ɪniːkxɑːh]: a female speaker.

verbal, the morphological structure of the verb is likely to be a major factor in the characterization of the sound patterns that emerge in the lexicon. In this way, the phonetic characteristics of the Navajo language are in the verbal patterns, not in the phoneme inventory. A discussion of these distributional asymmetries will be taken up in the chapters on morphology (Chapter 2), phonology (Chapter 3) and timing and duration (Chapter 4).

Let me give one example. The boundary between the final and penult syllables is a discernable juncture in Navajo speech. Note the spectrogram in Figure 3. This is a spectrogram of the utterance *ch'íniikááh* [tʃ'ɪniːkxɑːh] 'they go out', spoken by a female. Several characteristic aspects of Navajo speech are demonstrated in this spectrogram, including the sharp onset and offset of consonant and vowel articulations, discussed in detail Chapters 4 and 5. Relevant to the present discussion, note the final syllable as marked by the arrow. This syllable makes up nearly half the duration of the word. This is the stem, the unique position of the consonantal contrasts. The onset of this syllable is the aspirated velar stop *k* [kx]; it is quite prominent in the signal. This juncture is the only place in the word where consonant clusters consistently appear. The juncture is a striking aspect of the speech signal, confirmed by the fact that, if speakers paused in the pronunciation of words in this dataset, they paused at this juncture. There were no instances of pauses anywhere else in the verb word. The nature of the stem prominence and the relationship of the stem to the pre-stem domains are questions a phonetic study of the sound system must address. For this reason, I begin with an outline of the verbal morphology in Chapter 2, followed by a chapter on the phonology of the Navajo language, which is based on the morphological model and lays out the clearly phonologically driven processes in Navajo, such as consonant harmony.

Chapter 4 describes the timing and duration properties of the verb, through an investigation of the three domains within the verb and the aspects of the sounds that occur within the domains. Finally, in Chapter 5, we take up a study of the spectral qualities of the phonemes.

A goal of this study is to provide a baseline study of the sound system of Navajo as a foundation for a broader, more in-depth study of the language. Understanding the effects of the asymmetrical distribution patterns may help to develop research questions that address the lexicon in Athabaskan, and in languages that have rich inflectional morphologies which are likely to share some of these distributional properties.

1.4 THE YOUNG AND MORGAN GRAMMARS

The Young and Morgan grammars and dictionaries (Young and Morgan 1943, 1980, 1987, 1992, Young 2000) are the primary reference grammars for Navajo. They represent sixty years of work on the Navajo language by this team. The grammars contain a wealth of explicit information on the structure of the language. They lay out in detail the morphology of Navajo; each morpheme is discussed separately, and they provide examples of sentences, which were collected, not constructed, and thus represent language use.

I will use the 1987 version of Young and Morgan as the standard reference for the morpheme glosses and examples used in this book unless otherwise noted. I will refer to *The Navajo Language* as a 'grammar' for convenience. The Young and Morgan 1980 and 1987 grammars are divided into two sections, with separate numbering. The first section is a grammar, followed by a dictionary where Navajo word forms are listed alphabetically. I will indicate reference to these sections in the glosses as 'g' (grammar) or 'd' (dictionary), i.e. 'Young and Morgan 1987:g336', or 'Young and Morgan 1987:d220'.

One of the most important contributions of the grammar to Navajo studies and to linguistic research is the paradigm system used in the grammar. The dictionaries are word-based; that is, the dictionary entries are listed as fully inflected words and the entries are cross-referenced (by a page number in parenthesis in the middle margin) to the conjugational paradigms that they are associated to.

Throughout the grammar, as a foundation to word formation, YM have provided extensive and explicit paradigms and conjugations in both the grammar and the dictionary sections. The paradigms are the basis of word formation in YM, not morphemes, as they clearly state (:g200). The paradigms are cross-referenced to associated dictionary entries and they can be broken down into their morphemic structure, and the morphemes can located in both the grammar and the dictionary sections. While the paradigms are the basis of word formation, the morphemes are the instruments for examining the morpho-syntactic aspects of the verb in the grammar section, such as the aspectual system (g164-189), the behavior of the agreement markers (g64-80) or the classifiers (g117-127). Since the Athabaskan languages have a highly productive and complex morphology, the structure of the YM grammar is worthy of study for anyone interested in Athabaskan. Chapter 6 is a tutorial on the structure of the YM grammar. It primarily addresses the use of the paradigms and is meant to be used in conjunction with the 1987 version of *The Navajo Language.*

1.5   THE CONVENTIONS USED IN THE BOOK

I have adopted several transcription conventions from Young and Morgan. First, I have adopted the conventional Athabaskan terms 'disjunct' 'conjunct' and 'stem' to refer to the three major domains in the word. The structure of the verb and the internal structure of the domains is explained in Chapter 2 on morphology. I use the conventional symbol '#' to mark the boundary between the disjunct and conjunct domains.

An example gloss is given in (2). The first line is the Navajo word given in the orthography. The final line is the translation of this word with a reference to the page number in YM 1987 where the form can be found. Recall the 'd' and 'g' (as in 'YM d223') refer to the dictionary and grammar sections of *The Navajo Language,* which have separate numbering.Thus every word in this book can be located in the grammar and, for most words, the associated paradigms can also be located.

(2)   yis dzį́į́s
       [ish   ] [ø   dzį́į́s   ]
       [øimp/1s] ['cl' drag, tow:imp]
       [VII/VIII] [IX   X   ]
       [Aux   ] [Verb   ]
       'I'm dragging or towing it along' (YM:d775)[4]

The morpheme-by-morpheme glosses are given in the second line, and the transliteration of those glosses, adapted from those given in Young and Morgan, are listed in the next line. The fourth line indicates the position class of the morpheme in the gloss for reference to morph-syntactic information, and the fifth line indicates the domain that morpheme is associated with. In this book I have assumed Young and Morgan's strategy of building the words from the Base Paradigms. This is reflected in the glosses; these Base Paradigm forms are portmanteaus of Pos VII and VIII and identified as to their conjugation such as ø-imperfective, n-perfective, or optative. In example (2) the *ish* in the second line is the 1st person singular form of the ø imperfective conjugation (øimp/1s, Pos. VII/VIII), as listed in YM (g200). I also assume domain boundaries that are slightly different from the usual view of the position class template, as discussed in Chapter 2. The glosses put the morpheme *ish* (øimp/1s) at the right edge of a domain called Aux. The classifier prefix, 'cl', is included with the verb stem in the Verb domain. The core verb, the basic or minimal verb, contains a form from one of the Base Paradigms (Pos. VII/VIII), and a verb unit, which is a classifier (Pos. IX and which may be null, as above) and a verb stem (Pos. X).

Using the dictionary entries and the paradigms, cross references can be made to the stem and root appendix (g318-56) and the Base Paradigm charts (g200-01) and the Model Paradigm charts (g206-256). The dictionary entries also provide glosses of all the morphemes found in an entry, outside the obligatory morphemes of the core verb. The structure of the 1987 grammar is discussed in detail in Chapter 6. The morpheme by morpheme glosses and transliterations given in the book reflect the glosses and paradigms of the Young and Morgan grammar.

I also adopt the usage of the terms 'stem' and 'root' from Young and Morgan. A 'root' is an abstraction over the surface forms of a stem (Hardy 1969). The verb stems are inflected for aspect, and this inflection changes the shape of the stem. Roots are a means of talking about the stems independent of their aspect. Young and Morgan list these roots/stems in their imperfective reflex in the Root / Theme / Stem appendix (g352). I adopt the YM convention of using caps to signify the verb 'root' morpheme as such: -YóóD (Also note that the fricative and glide-initial stems are listed in their voiced reflex, since voicing is not phonemic in stems[5].). The term 'stems sets' refers to the related set of reflexes of this root. For instance, one stem set for the root -YóóD is the set: -yóód (imperfective), yo' (repetitive), yood (perfective), yoł (future), yóód (optative). The stem sets are usually associated with a classifier as indicated in the dictionary. The relationship between the shape of a stem and its various aspectual realizations is not well understood, but the most complete discussion of the stem allomorphy can be found in Hardy (1969). A list of all the Navajo roots and their various stem reflexes and their patterns of association to the classifiers, which YM (g302) number around 8700, can be found in the root/stem dictionary.

1.6   METHODS AND DATA SETS

The study is based on several sets of recordings and studies made over nine years, of Navajo speakers reciting specially prepared wordlists that exemplify the sound contrasts and prosody of Navajo. The recordings used in this monograph are grouped into three main data sets: the first made in 1992, a second set in 1995, and a third set in January 2001. The primary set used in this study is the January 2001 set. The 1992 data set was used in the analysis of the first vowel study and in the first study of the stop consonants of the verb stem. The 1995 recordings were made on the reservation, in Kayenta, Arizona and on Navajo Mountain. This fieldwork associated with this data set was accomplished under the direction of Martha Austin-Garrison of Diné College. The 2001 work was accomplished under the direction of Ms. Austin-Garrison and Anthony Goldtooth Sr. of Diné College. Ms. Austin-Garrison was present at all the recording sessions reported on in this monograph, and she was the primary consultant on this project. The speakers in all these studies, with the exception of the Navajo Mountain recordings, were educated native speakers of Navajo, who live on the reservation and use Navajo daily; they were all bilingual. Speakers were recorded while repeating a word list that was developed to illustrate various aspects of the sound system. The first set of recordings was made in a classroom at Navajo Community College, Shiprock, New Mexico, in April 1992 in conjunction with Peter Ladefoged and Helen George of UCLA and Clay Slate of Diné College.

The first two word lists were developed to illustrate the phonemic contrasts; these were primarily prefix-noun combinations. The standard means of finding was used. We used the prefix *bi-* 3rd singular pronoun and a simple noun stem to provide as stable a context as possible for the sounds we wished to examine. An example is *bi + taa': bitaa'*, 'his father'. In this way, all the consonants were intervocalic, preceded by the orthographic high front vowel *i*. Since the language does not lend itself to the construction of minimal pairs, the vowel contrasts were gathered from stems that had those contrasts; we were not able to maintain a unique stem-initial consonant in the dataset. In the first recording, we asked speakers to repeat items in isolation and in a frame sentence, but speakers treated the tokens in frame sentences as they did isolation items, so this practice was discontinued. In general speakers disliked repeating tokens, finding the repetition awkward and tending to make speakers self conscious. In later recordings, I abandoned this technique as counterproductive. The third word list was constructed to illustrate tonal contrasts within the verb word, and was used in the tone studies (McDonough 1999, 2002), as well in as the recordings of the dataset for the present study. The fourth world list was constructed to illustrate the sounds that occurred in the conjunct and disjunct domains; this is also a verb list. The final list was constructed to demonstrate three kinds of constructions: declarative, focus and yes/no questions. These are short utterances in which a statement is followed by either a yes/no question or a focus construction.

All the word lists were developed and checked for accuracy and acceptability by Martha Austin-Garrison prior to fieldwork. In the recording sessions, items which a speaker found problematic were not used.

A small study of monolingual speakers was conducted with Martha Austin-Garrison in the Navajo Mountain area of the reservation in Arizona west of Monument National Park. The speakers were recorded one-on-one, reciting a list of words after Ms. Austin-Garrison who speaks this dialect. The speakers were all in their 60's and 70's, none had received a western education and were, for the greater part, unfamiliar with the orthography of Navajo. They were recorded at their homes using a Marantz PMD 340 cassette tape recorder with a Sony directional microphone. This data from this study is discussed in the context of the vowel spaces in Chapter 5.

The recordings made in January 2001 make up the primary data of this study. These were made in a classroom at Diné College, Shiprock, at the Navajo Education Center, with the help of Martha Austin-Garrison and Anthony Goldtooth, Sr.. Because the traditional Navajo community is primarily an oral culture, we wanted to provide the subjects with oral prompts, rather than written text. To this end, we recorded Ms. Austin-Garrison while we were discussing and reading the lists, using a Tascam portable DAT recorder. The DAT tape was then digitalized into a Mac Powerbook G3, using SoundEdit 16. A master file was made from the best tokens on the tape. The tokens were organized into lists and split into 5 sound files, which were presented to the subjects. Silences of 1000 ms were spliced between tokens to give speakers adequate time to repeat the token after hearing the prompt. These 5 soundfiles were presented as prompts in individual recording sessions to 16 native Navajo speakers from the Mac powerbook. The subjects were asked to repeat the token after the prompt. Speakers wore a Shure head-mounted microphone attached to the DAT recorder and we were able to stop the recordings at any time. The recording sessions lasted about 20-30 minutes.

At the University of Rochester, the DAT tapes were digitalized and burned directly onto CD's in a professional recording studio at the Eastman School of Music. The files were then transferred to .aiff files and they were segmented and analyzed using Praat 4.0 on a Mac G4 in the speech lab in the Department of Linguistics. The word lists and glosses are listed in Appendix 1. The word lists and recording sessions are discussed briefly again in the methodology sections of Chapters 4 (Duration and Timing) and 5 (Spectral Analyses) for clarification purposes.

1.7   OUTLINE OF THE BOOK

The view of phonetics and phonetic description taken in this work is slightly different than the one practiced by phoneticians who are primarily interested in particular aspects of the segmental or prosodic system. The goal of this work is to provide a picture of the system as whole, and I have made decisions on what to include based on a desire to provide an overview of what I understand of the system. There are many omissions, in part due to time and space limitations, and in part due to the scope limitations of a single research study. There are blatant omissions. I have not included, for instance, a significant discussion of tone, because preliminary studies have been done outside this book (deJong and McDonough 1992, McDonough 2000, McDonough 2002) and a more detailed investigation is a monograph size study in itself. An investigation of the tonal prosody across Athabaskan is likely to be essential in understanding the organization of the lexicon and variation across the Athabaskan languages. Preliminary investigation of utterance-level tonal prosody, for instance, suggests that there is a close relationship between the syntactic properties of the morphology and its tonal typology. If these features change across the language family, it's likely that the tonal prosody will be affected (Hale et. al. 2001, McDonough 2002). In the chapter on the spectral analyses I have limited the discussion to the major properties of the phonemic system, the spectral properties of the fricatives and vowels. I have not included, for example, a study of the stops bursts, or the effect of the preceding consonant on the vowel formants, though these are important aspects of these sounds.

The book is constructed as follows: Chapter 2 discusses the morphological structure of the verb; Chapter 3 is an overview of the primary phonological processes in the grammar as they are relevant to the sound contrasts and phonotactics. These chapter lay the foundation for a discussion of the phonetics of Navajo. Chapter 4 is a report on an investigation of the timing and duration facts in the verb word; Chapter 5 discusses the spectral aspects of the sounds, concentrating on the fricatives and the vowel system. Chapter 6 is a discussion of the structure of the 1987 Young and Morgan grammar. This chapter is written to stand independent from the rest of the book; it is intended at a tutorial on *The Navajo Language*. Chapter 7 is a summary chapter.

---

[1] Indeed, Edward Sapir and P. E. Goddard, working on Athabaskan at the turn of the last century, recognized the need for instrumental phonetic documentation and involved themselves in collecting instrumental data in the field (Goddard 1904, 1905, Goddard and Sapir 1907, Sapir 1938). In a study of Hupa, Gordon (1996), for instance, makes reference to palatographic studies that were done on Hupa by Goddard in 1907, 90 years previously.

[2] The optimal length of a verb in Navajo bears discussion, though the means of answering it are presently not available. The impressive complexity of the template may lead to an assumption that the verb words may be quite long. But doesn't seems to be the case. The verbs are usually not more than three or four syllables long, perhaps shorter in real discourse, as Navajo linguists have suggested (Willie p.c.). In the development of the wordlist, for instance, the longest conjunct domain I as able to elicit was three syllables long. When I pressed my consultants, they conceded to my requests for longer verbs by giving me longer disjunct domains. I have not seen this discussed in the literature on Athabaskan, I have not investigated this matter, and the YM grammar can't be used for frequency counts, but if three syllables is the longest conjunct domain then this may be a causal factor in the apparent compression of morphemes in conjunct domain. While the compression may be phonologically motivated, a three syllable conjunct constraint is not obviously so. These questions await the development of digital language corpora for Navajo.

[3] This count is based on the CD version of the dictionary, the Lockard CD (1999).

[4] The translations are as close as possible to the ones given in YM. This means that sometimes an infintive translation of the verb is given, though all the Navajo verbs are

marked for person and number. Use of the infinitive also bypasses the problem of translating the various Navajo Modes into the English tense system.

[5] Voicing is not a feature of contrast for fricatives in the onset of stems, which is the position of the phonemes in Athabaskan. It does show up as contrastive in the coda of the Aux and Verb stems, in both cases it also carries morphological or grammatical meaning. For example *mááz* is the perfective form of the verb stem *Máás* 'roll', and *-(y)iz* is the 3[rd]s form of the s-perfective (ø/ł) (vs. *–(ji)s* 3[rd]s of the s-perfective (d/l)). See YM:337g and 201g for examples. See also the discussion of the voicing in fricatives in Chapter 5.2.

Chapter 2

MORPHOLOGY

2.0 INTRODUCTION

The Athabaskan verb can stand alone as a proposition; it is capable of denoting an event. The role of the verbal morphology is to provide the means for this task. It does so with a rich lexicon of grammatical, inflectional and adverbial morphemes and agreement markers, a structure that supports the interpretation of these morphemes, and a word formation system that allows the verb to be constructed in maximally simple and productive ways. The structure of the Athabaskan verb has been under discussion for over one hundred years. Morice's (1932) grammar of Carrier (Dakelh) observed that, despite the complexity of the morphology, the verbs were made up of two core parts, a verb part and a tense and subject part. Sapir established a slot-and-filler template to describe the ordering of the verbal morphemes, versions of which are in common use today. But he also observed that investigation of the verbal morphology would likely prove the verb to be considerably more 'analytic' than his complex template indicated; he suggested the verb word fell apart easily and would prove to be made up of 'little verbs' (Sapir 1925).

A commonly-used model of Athabaskan morphology is a version of the Sapir slot-and-filler or 'position class' template. This template has been used for two distinct and often conflicting purposes. One is for the description of the morphemes in the verb and their order, without respect to their status in the grammar. In this, the template has proven to be a valuable tool for comparative Athabaskan and Dine studies. It has helped advanced our understanding of the language family and this morphological type. The second purpose is as a word formation device and structure for interpretation. In this it has been less successful, primarily because, used as a formal model, the template represents an odd morphological type, and, particular to the Athabaskan case, it does not allow us to see the verbal paradigms in a language family whose verbal morphology is indisputably inflectional and paradigmatic. The position class template makes no distinction between morphemes that are quite abstract, such as the conjugation markers, and those that are paired with sound, such as the object markers, yet these distinction are likely to have an effect on paradigm

17

building and word formation. In addition, the positions are ad hoc. They do not have formal status in morphology; the template is essentially a prosthesis used to support morpheme ordering, which it does well. As a word formation device, however, the template requires that elaborate theoretical and procedural adjustments be invented to handle it, mainly because the linear order of positions cannot be used as a concatenation order and because the concatenation of template morphemes often requires extensive rewrite rules (Hargus 1987, Kari 1992).

In this chapter I will outline an alternate model of the morphological structure in Navajo called the bipartite model. It is a principled morphological model of paradigm concatenation, it is simple, and it is tied closely to the word formation strategies used in Young and Morgan.

2.1   ATHABASKAN WORD STRUCTURE

The following examples of Navajo verbs exemplify two important characteristics of their structure. Example (1) shows that the minimal verb is two syllables long and the language is 'prefixal': the verb stem is the final syllable in the word, preceded by a pre-stem complex. The second example shows that the pre-stem material can be quite complex. The glosses are discussed in Section 2.3.1 below[1].

(1)   yish cha
    [(y)ish   ] [ø   cha   ]
    [øimp/1s] ['cl' 'cry']
    [VII/VIII] [IX X (stem)]
    [Aux   ] [Verb   ]
    'I cry' (YM87:d779)

(2)   bíbiniis sįįh
    bí   # [bi ni   (y)i (i)sh   ] [ł   zįįh   ]
    against # [3o termin trans Øimp/1s] [trans 'stand']
    I   [V VI   VI   VII/VIII] [IX X (stem)]
     D # [Aux   ] [Verb   ]
    'I lean him against it, in a standing position' (YM87:d169)

First, note that there are three major domains in the verb, the disjunct (D), conjunct (or Aux, see discussion below) and verb stem (Verb) domains, although not all verbs have disjunct morphemes. The two syllables in (1) represent a core verb, with the minimal morphosyntactic specification. The foundation of the verb is the verb stem (*cha* 'cry' in (1) above), the rightmost element in the verb, and it is a content morpheme. The syllable to its left in (1) is comprised of morphemes indicating mode and subject (person and number). This morpheme (*yish*) corresponds to the 1st person singular form of the Mode conjugation, ø-imperfective. These morphemes are in positions VII and VIII in Young and Morgan's version of the position class template (1987:g37-8) (see Section 2.2). Example (2) has a more complex morphemic structure, as indicated by the glosses. Taken together, these morphemes indicate direction, valency, subject and object marking as well as several aspectual properties of the proposition, in addition to the base meaning of the verb stem -zįįh 'stand'. The nature of this verbal construction, and its morphemic structure in general, is the concern of this chapter.

I assume a model in which the verb is a simple compound of two components, Aux and Verb, preceded by a set of proclitics ('D' or disjunct), as in (3). This is termed the bipartite model. In this view, the Athabaskan 'conjunct' domain is the auxiliary (Aux), as indicated. Arguments for this structure can be found in McDonough 1990, 1996, 2000a, 2000b.

(3)   [Proclitics # [AGR [af - stem]$_{Aux}$ [af - stem   ]$_{Verb}$]$_{Verb\ Word}$
         Disjunct # [Conjunct   ] [Verb Stem]
            D   # [Aux   ] [Verb   ]

In this view, each of the two syntactic domains, Aux and Verb, has a morpheme from the category 'stem' as a head. Affixation is to the stem within a domain. The Aux stem corresponds to a form from one of the 16 primary conjugations of Young and Morgan's Base Paradigms (YM 1987:200-01). These conjugations mark the aspectual modes in Navajo, four imperfective modes (ø-, ni- si-, and yi- imperfectives) and eight corresponding perfective modes (two perfective for each imperfective, see YM:g200 for discussion), and a repetitive, progressive, optative and future mode. The modes are marked for person and number (singular and dual). Thus (y)ish is the 1st singular form of the ø imperfective mode (øimp/1st). The Aux stem and the Verb stem are the two core parts of the verb; they are paradigmatic in nature and they constitute the minimal morphosyntactic specification of a verb in Athabaskan.

In addition to the Aux stem, the Aux domain contains two sets of prefixes: the 'Qualifier' prefixes, which arguably play an aspectual role in the grammar, conditioning the event semantics of the verb (Sussman and McDonough 2003, Smith 2000), and also the Agreement markers of Pos IV and V in the position class template. The Verb domain has a verb stem as a head and is prefixed by the 'classifiers', which are valence or voice markers (The name classifier is a source of misunderstanding to those unfamiliar with Athabaskan terminology. These morphemes are misnamed; they are not classifying or gender morphemes but rather a set of valence or voice markers.). In the template these 'classifiers' are part of the conjunct prefix domain; in the bipartite model, these prefixes form a unit with the verb stem, called a 'verb unit', and this unit comprises the Verb domain. The resulting compound structure is a syntactically valid entity. We will discuss this model and its relationship to the position class template in section 2.3.1.

Despite the complexity of Athabaskan morphology and the various formalisms used to model it, there are several uncontroversial aspects to the Athabaskan verb. It is generally agreed that it is minimally bisyllabic, with a verb stem as its rightmost morpheme; the verbal structure is primarily prefixal, as we see in the schema in (3). Finally, as noted, the verb contains sufficient inflection to build a proposition. What is controversial is the internal structure of the domains of the verb, and the status of its morphemes. This controversy is exemplified by the model used to represent the verb, the relationship between the morphosyntax, morphophonology and prosody, and the nature of morpheme concatenation and word formation.

2.2   THE POSITION CLASS TEMPLATE

Several, often conflicting, models of Athabaskan verbal morphology exist (Morice 1932, Sapir-Hoijer 1967, Kari 1976, 1990, 1992, McDonough 1990, 2000a, 2000b, Halpern 1992, Hargus 1987, 1994, Randoja 1989, Rice 1989, 2000). Generally, however, a version of the 'slot-and-filler' or 'position class' template is used as a basis of word formation in the current literature on Athabaskan.

A 'slot-and-filler' or 'position class' template is a morphology that consists of slots or positions into which morphemes are plugged; a morpheme is assigned to a particular position based on its distribution with respect to other morphemes. The slots are numbered (in Athabaskan, from left to right using roman numerals by convention), and they do the work of keeping the morphemes ordered. Thus subject marking (position VIII) is to the right of the Mode (position VII in the template) because subject marking always appears between the Mode and the stem.

Unfortunately, the ordering template doesn't work well as a model of concatenation. In Kari's (1992) discussion of Athabaskan word formation based on the template, the verb requires at least 8 cycles in the phonology, and, since not every verb requires every cycle, the cycles themselves are a horizontal extension of the template, invoked to support the discontinuous concatenation imposed by the template. Kari (1992:34) , in fact, admits that the concatenation model is not fully functional. For instance, in this model the subject morpheme (VIII) is inserted several levels after the Mode (VII) morpheme, but must combine with it in paradigmatic (i.e. opaque) ways. In this way, the template slots are a prosthesis; position classes are only used when other more common or principled means of ordering fail (for discussion of the status of position classes in the grammar see Simpson and Withgott 1989, Stump 1992, McDonough 2000a). It is a common but implicit assumption of those who use the template as a base of word formation that the properties of the template are the properties of

Athabaskan word formation (Kari 1992, Faltz 2000, Rice 2000). I contest this assumption: the properties of the template model can be examined independently of the properties of the verb; if it doesn't work well, other models can be developed.

In the version of the template that Young and Morgan provide in their 1987 grammar (YM87:g37-38), the template has seventeen positions (including subpositions) divided into 3 domains, the disjunct, conjunct and stem respectively. The Young and Morgan template is provided in Table 6.

Table 6 The 'position class' template of Young and Morgan (YM87:g37-38). (For a list of the morphemes assigned to each slot see Young and Morgan.)

0	I					II	III	IV	V	VI			VII	VIII	IX	X
	a	b	c	d	e					a	b	c				

KEY (from left to right):

0	*Direct object of postposition.* *Possessive prefix with nouns.*	
Ia	Null postposition	
Ib	Adverbial – Thematic ('postpositional stems')	
Ic	(Reflexive)	**Disjunct**
Id	(Reversionary)	
Ie	(Semeliterative)	
II	(Iterative)	
III	(Distributive Plural)	

IV	Direct Object Pronouns	
V	Deictic Subject Pronouns	
VIa	Adverbial – Thematic	
VIb	Adverbial – Thematic	**Conjunct**
VIc	Transitional / Semelfactive Aspect markers	
VII	Modal - Aspectival Conjugation markers	
VIII	Subject Pronouns	
IX	'Classifier'	

X	Stem	**Stem**

The classifications provided for each of the slots are listed in the table as they are in Young and Morgan. All the morphemes in the position classes but the rightmost one are called prefixes. The position classes are constructed to represent the distribution of morphemes. Some morphemes are necessary to the word; they represent the minimum morphosyntactic represent that a fully infected verb form requires. These are the rightmost morphemes, positions VII, VIII, IX and X, the Mode, subject, 'classifier' and verb stem respectively, the core verb. The rest of the positions represent morphemes which are not essential. We will discuss the make-up of each of the major domains in sections 2.4, 2.5, and 2.6. For a full discussion of the morphemes in the template, I refer the reader to the sections in Young and Morgan on the template morphemes (g206-250) and the sections on aspect (g164-189) and on the Base and Extended Paradigms (g200-01), as well as the general literature on Athabaskan languages, such as Platero and Fernald (2002), Rice (2000), Jelinek (1989), Willie and Jelinek (2000), Thompson (1993), Faltz (2000), and Gunlogson (2001).

As Navajo is indisputably an inflectional language, paradigms are an important part of the verbal structure. Identifying them and delineating their role in word formation is essential to understanding the structure of the verb. In Young and Morgan's *The Navajo Language* (1980, 1987), the unequivocal basis of all word formation are inflectional paradigms. Both the dictionary and grammar sections are filled with explicit and careful verbal paradigms and instructions on how to combine them into words. Although Young and Morgan provide a template-based morpheme analysis (g39-139), they use the template only as a reference, not as a word formation device. Instead, two main paradigms act as the base of word formation in YM: the Base Paradigms or mode conjugations, and the verb stem sets. These two paradigm sets have distinct properties and they are laid out in *The Navajo Language* (1987) in Appendices I and V. Appendix I introduces and lists the 16 basic mode conjugations, Appendix V lists the verb stem sets. As for their beliefs about word formation in Navajo, Young and Morgan write explicitly: "The 16 Base and Extended Base Paradigms constitute the foundation upon which all verb bases are conjugated." (g200). These Base Paradigms are the Aux stems, the head of the Aux domain in the bipartite model. They are essentially portmanteaus of position VII (Mode) and VIII (subject) (See Chapter 6 for further discussion of the structure of the 1987 *The Navajo Language* and their use of paradigms in word formation.).

The 'slot-and-filler' or position class template reduces paradigmatic inflection to a problem of morpheme concatenation, and it does not separate out paradigm building from more transparent prefix attachment. I've adopted a simpler model of verbal structure in this monograph, the bipartite structure, on the reasonable assumption that difficult structures are likely to be reanalyzed by language learners into simpler ones over time. If we can build the verb from simple, more widely found and validated grammatical units, then the more complex constructions are likely to be superfluous. So we will begin with a parsimonious structure and build complexity into it only when forced to.

My aim is not to dismiss the Athabaskan template, which is an indisputable and valuable tool of analysis, but to offer a simpler model drawn from language internal evidence that reflects the paradigmatic and inflectional aspects of the verb and can be used to represent a language community's knowledge of structure. In the next sections, the major divisions in the verb will be outlined, the differences between the template and the bipartite model will be briefly discussed for reference, and the terminology in use in the Athabaskan literature will be defined.

2.3 THE ATHABASKAN VERB

There are three well established domains in the Athabaskan verb (Sapir-Hoijer 1967, Kari 1989, 1976): the disjunct (D), conjunct (Aux) and Verb stem (Verb). The three groups are marked in the rightmost column in the key to the positions in Table 6. In (4) is a schema of the three domains, in the second line are the names assigned to these domains by the bipartite model.

(4)   Disjunct # [Conjunct] [Verb Stem]
          D   # [Aux   ] [Verb   ]

Each of these domains has properties that distinguish it from the other domains in the word. The leftmost domain (D) contains a group of morphemes with clitic-like properties. The domain is optional in the sense that all the morphemes in this domain are optional, though subcategorization constraints on these morphemes may be present in some constructions. The boundary between the disjunct and conjunct domains is typographically marked with a '#' in the morpheme glosses, a convention in the Athabaskan literature which we will observe in this book. This boundary marks a well documented domain edge for morphophonemic rules (Sapir-Hoijer 1967, Kari 1976, Young and Morgan 1980, 1987); I refer the reader to these works for discussion. The middle domain is the conjunct or Aux domain, and the rightmost domain is the verb. The core verb contains morphemes from the conjunct and stem domains in the ways discussed in the following sections.

2.3.1 The Bipartite Model

As noted, I will assume a model of the Navajo verb argued for in McDonough (1990, 2000a, 2000b), called the bipartite model. In this model the core verb is a compound of two syntactic units, an Aux and a Verb. Each unit is rightheaded and has a base which belongs to the morphological category 'stem'. The core verb is represented in (5), with the position classes beneath for reference. Note that there is a set of prefixes for each base; these are the Qualifiers (Kari's (1990) term for the Aspect morphemes of pos VI) and 'classifier'[2] prefixes (pos IX) respectively. An additional set of AGR prefixes can be attached to the compound, as in (6). These are the object agreement and 'deictic subject' markers of pos IV and V. Finally the

pro-clitic 'disjunct' group is to the left in (7), containing positions III and
leftward in the template. The result is a grammatical word.

(5)   [(af) Base   ]$_{Aux}$ [(af) Base]$_{Verb}$
        [VI VII/VIII]   [IX X   ]
        [Aux   ]   [Verb   ]

(6)   [(AGR (af) Base   ]$_{Aux}$ [(af) Base]$_{Verb}$
        [IV/V VI VII/VIII]   [IX X   ]
        [Aux   ]   [Verb   ]

(7)   [Proclitics # [(AGR (af) Base   ]$_{Aux}$ [(af) Base]$_{Verb}$]$_{Verb}$
             00-III # [IV/V VI VII/VIII]   [IX X   ]
                 D   # [Aux   ]   [Verb   ]

The examples below illustrate the structure of the verb. The second and
third lines in the examples are the morpheme-by-morpheme glosses and
morpheme transliterations. The fourth line is the alignment of the template
position classes to the bipartite model for reference; the final line is the
domain division: D, Aux or Verb. (8) is an example of the minimal verb,
corresponding to (5) above. It's comprised of the two stems, Aux *yish*
(øimp/1st) and Verb *dzíís*, with no prefixes (the 'classifier' is null.). The
form *yish* is the 1st singular form of the ø-imperfective mode paradigm
(øimp/1st) (YM:g200), and the verb stem is an imperfective alternant of the
root *DZiiS*^{3} 'drag, pull, tow' (YM:g326). These two parts of the verb must
agree in mode; in this example they are both in the imperfective mode. (9)
is an example that also corresponds to (5) above, but both stems have
prefixes, the Qualifier (*di-* 'inceptive' (YM:d333)) and 'classifier' (*ł-*)
prefixes respectively.

(8)   yis dzíís
        [(y)ish   ] [ø   dzíís   ]
        [øimp/1s] ['cl'   drag, tow:imp]
        [VII/VIII] [IX   X   ]
        [Aux   ] [Verb   ]
        'I'm dragging or towing it along' (YM:d775)

(9)   dish ch'ą́ą́ł
        [d(i) ish   ] [ł   ch'ą́ą́ł   ]
        [Qu- øimp/1s] ['cl' hang suspended from a rope:imp]
        [VI VII/VIII] [IX   X   ]
        [Aux   ] [Verb   ]
        'I start down (using a rope)' (YM:d334)

The example in (10) corresponds to (6) above: the Aux stem is *nish*, the n-imperfective conjugation 1st singular (YM:g200), and the prefix to the Aux is the Agr prefix, the 3rds object pronoun *ho* (a 3rd person marker for animate objects or for space, area, or the "impersonal" YM:g66*).* There is no qualifier prefix in this example. In (11), which corresponds to the structure indicated in (7) above, *bí* 'against' is a disjunct morpheme, and we see the two obligatory stems, the Aux *(y)ish* (øimp/1st) and the Verb *sįįh* with the classifier prefix *ł-*. The Aux stem, *(y)ish,* here shows the consonant harmony alternation *(y)is*. There are also two "Qualifier' (position VI) morphemes in the Aux domain, the terminative *ni* and *(y)i*^{4}- a combination which YM (:g187, d169) glosses as the transitional marker. Finally, at the left of the conjunct domain, the 3rd singular object marker *bi*.

(10) honish łįįh
     [ho nish   ] [ø   łįįh   ]
     [3s nimp/1s] ['cl' 'come, exist':imp]
     [IV VII/VIII] [IX X   ]
     [Aux   ] [Verb   ]
     'I appear, arrive' (YM87:d456)

(11) bíbiniis sįįh
     bí   # [bi n(i) (y)i (y)ish   ] [ł   sįįh   ]
     'against' # [3o term trans øimp/1s] ['cl' 'stand':imp]
     Ib   [V VI   VI   VII/VIII] [IX X   ]
         D   # [Aux   ] [Verb   ]
     'I lean him standing against it' (YM87:d169)

(12) haséł báąz
     ha   # [sé   ] [ł   báąz   ]
     'up out' # [s-imp/1s] ['cl' 'handle hooplike object':perf]
     Ib   [VII/VIII] [IX X   ]
         D   # [Aux] [Verb   ]
     'I drove it up' (YM:d429)

In (12) is an example with a disjunct prefix *ha*, 'up, out' (YM:g37), and a more basic Aux and Verb compound; the Aux consists of an Aux stem in the 1st singular form of the s-perfective conjugation *sé*; and the Verb is the stem *báąz* 'hooplike object' and a 'cl' *ł-*, the combination *ł-báąz* means 'move by rolling a hooplike object' (YM:g319). For a full discussion of these morphemes, with more examples, the reader may refer to Young and Morgan as indicated in the glosses[5].

2.4   THE DISJUNCT DOMAIN

The leftmost domain in the verb is the disjunct domain. YM refer to disjunct morphemes as "less tightly bound" components of the verb group (YM:g39) and state that these morphemes are "loosely integrated" into the verb complex, referring to the fact that they often appear as independent elements. They have a larger inventory of phonemes than the conjunct morphemes, including tonal contrasts, and their phonetic properties reflect their non-prefix status, though most of the variation is in the morphemes of pos Ib, the 'postpositional stems'. Examples of these are listed in (13).

(13)   na-   'around about'
        ch'í-   'out horizontally'
        'a-   'away out of sight'
        ha-   'up and out (as from a hole)'
        dzídza-   'into the fire'
        ta-   'into water'
        ni-   'cessative-terminative'

This domain contains a distributive plural and iterative marker and indirect object markers. Indirect object morphemes appear at the left edge of this domain, as in (14), for example.

(14)   bik'iish tłíísh
        bi k'i # [(y)i   (y)ish   ] [ø   tłish   ]
        3rd 'on' # [Trans øimp/1s] ['cl' 'move independently through the air']
           D   # [Aux   ] [Verb   ]
        I fell on it' (YM:d220)

When there are differences in opinion about the number and kind of slots in the Athabaskan template, disagreements are usually about the slots that occur at the left edge of the word. Some studies have indicated that the left edge of this domain may be less clearly marked as a boundary than the right edge of the word (McDonough and Willie 1998).

2.5   THE CONJUNCT OR AUXILIARY DOMAIN

In the bipartite view, the conjunct domain is auxiliary; its head is the Aux stem. The structure of this domain is one of the main points of difference between the template and bipartite model. In the template, this domain is flat and includes three position classes which are stipulated as obligatory in the verb. In the template view all the conjunct morphemes are prefixes. In Young and Morgan's 1987 template (Table 6) the conjunct domain contains six position classes (IV-IX), with three subclasses (VIa,

VIb, VIc). The three positions closest to the verb stem are obligatory, the *Mode* (VI), subject (VIII) and the classifier (XI) morphemes. In the bipartite view the classifiers are repositioned in the Verb domain. The other two obligatory morphemes, pos VII/VIII in the template, are the head of Aux, the Aux stem, a portmanteau of Mode and Subject. These forms constitute one of the two main paradigms in the verb. Young and Morgan call these the Base and Extended Paradigms.

2.5.1 Base and Extended Paradigms as the Head of Aux

YM (:g200-01) lists 16 *Base Paradigms* that constitute the 16 separate conjugations for these stems, 4 perfective, 8 perfective, an iterative, progressive, future and an optative. The forms are a portmanteau of positions VII/VIII. Table 7 gives the paradigms for the 1st -3rd person singular forms of the two s-perfective paradigms, paradigms that occur with the 'classifiers' /ø/ and /ł/, and those that appear with the /d/ and /l/ 'classifiers'. The forms are taken from the paradigm charts of Young and Morgan (g200). The term 'Extended Paradigm' requires comment. The 'Extended Paradigms' of the 'Base and Extended Paradigms' are extended by adding an AGR morpheme (object or 'deictic subject' pos V/VI) to the 3rd singular form of a Base conjugation. The Extended Paradigms as they are listed, then, include the 3rd person AGR morphemes they term 3o (object), 3s (space), and 3a (animate). They are presumably listed as part of the paradigm because the forms that arise from their concatenation are opaque.

Table 7 A partial Base paradigm for the two s-perfective Mode conjugations

	Person	ø - ł	d - l
	1	sé	sis
	2	síní	síní
	3	si	(yi)s
	3o	(y)iz	--
Extended	3a	jiz	jis
	3i	'az	'as
	3s	haz	has
	1dual	siid	siid
	2dual	soo	soo(h)

In (12) above the Aux stem is the 1st singular form from this paradigm. This form is a composite of the position VII and VIII *s* + *ish* in the template. The output of this concatenation is *sé*. I refer the reader to the discussion of Mode, aspect, subject and the Base Paradigms in the section on Mode and

Aspect (g144-189), and the section following the listing of the paradigms (g206-250).

In the bipartite view, forms from the cells of the Base conjugations carry the morphological specification 'stem' and are the head of the Aux. (15) shows a verb in the 1st person form of imperfective conjugation; the two stems agree in mode (imperfective). In (16), (17), and (18) the same verb is shown in three additional conjugations, repetitive, perfective and future; these forms were constructed from a paradigm chart in the YM dictionary (YM:d775). Note the change in the shape of the verb stem *tsid* 'pound', as its aspect changes:

(15) yis tsid
      [(y)ish   ] [ø   tsid   ]
      [øimp/1s] ['cl' 'pound':imp]
      [Aux   ] [Verb   ]
      'I pound it' (YM:d777)

(16) nás tsi' (R)
      ná   # [(y)ish   ] [ø   tsi'   ]
      iterative # [øimp/1s] ['cl' 'pound':rep]
            D   [Aux   ] [Verb   ]
            'I repeatedly pound it'

(17) yí tseed (P)
      [(y)í   ] [ø   tseed   ]
      [øperf/1s] ['cl' 'pound':perf]
      [Aux   ] [Verb   ]
      'I pounded it'

(18) dee tsił (F)
      [deesh   ] [ø   tsid   ]
      [future/1s] ['cl' 'pound':imp]
      [Aux   ] [Verb   ]
      'I'll pound it'

Evidence for the Aux morpheme's status as 'stem' is its position in the word and its phonotactics. These morphemes have the phonotactics of stem syllables, with long vowels and, crucially, coda consonants. Only stems have codas. The edge between the Aux and the Verb the single place in the word where consonant clusters appear, and it is a prominent boundary in the word[6].

2.5.2   Other Conjunct Morphemes

Outside the Aux stem, two other groups of morphemes are in the conjunct domain: the Qualifiers of position VIa, b, c, and the agreement markers of positions IV and V, as we've seen. All of their phonotactics are similar; they are primarily CV in shape and these prefixes have either the default vowel *i-* [ɪ] or they have a phonological variant of it. Also, the consonants in these prefixes are drawn from a reduced set of the phonemic contrasts; all manner and place features are neutralized. The set of conjunct consonants are *{d, s, sh, n, h, ', ł, j}*, with the later two [*ł, j*] appearing only in a small number of conjunct morphemes (See Young and Morgan 1987 :37-38 for the list of the conjunct morphemes, and Kari (1979) for an explicit discussion of the rules needed to produce the surface forms from the conjunct position classes.). Examples of these prefixes are in (11) above.

What is important to us in this study is that these two sets of morphemes, Agr and Qu, are prefixes on the Aux stem, they have a characteristic shape, *Ci-,* and the variants from this *Ci-* shape can be captured by phonological rules. Thus the morphemes of the Aux domain are: [AGR- Qu- stem].

2.6   THE VERB DOMAIN

In Navajo, the Verb domain is a single syllable long, the last syllable in the verb (barring nominalizing enclitics). The base of the Verb domain is the verb stem, and the 'classifiers' are prefixes to the verb stem. The stem has particular phonotactic properties: it is the single place in the word where the full set of consonantal and vocalic contrasts occur; the contrasts in the conjunct and disjunct domains are neutralized. The Aux stem and the Verb stem comprise the core verb and constitute the two main parts of the fully inflected grammatical word.

2.6.1   The Verb Stem

The verb stem is the main meaning unit in the verb. It is classificatory in the sense that the verb stem refers to properties that objects have in the world, such as round or flat. YM provides lists of verb stems in Appendices II through V (g251-356). Appendix V, the Root/ Stem / Theme list, is the principle stem appendix, listing the stems sets for Navajo verbs under the entries for a verb stem. A stem set is a list of the verb stems inflected for mode and associated to a particular aspect. The entries are capitalized by convention, and listed in their voiced, imperfective form. We can consider the capitalized form a root. Examples of entries are in (19). In (20) is an example of one series of stem alternations, or stem set, for the root *-ZÁÁS,* which becomes *ł+ ZÁÁS* (=sáás) in the 'Momentative' aspect.

(19)   *-JÁÁH*   move handle
                       (plural objects, usually small in size and large in number)
        -GHÁÁSH   to boil, bubble, shout, sleep
        -ZÁÁS   to dribble, strew, sprinkle

(20)   *sáás (I), *sas(R), *sas(P), *sas(F), *sáás (O) (ł) (Mom.)

These 'stem set' forms are paradigmatic in the sense that they appear in
a series of shapes that are marked for aspect (imperfective, repetitive,
perfective, future and optative, respectively). These shapes are listed in
Appendix V the Root/ Stem/ Theme list (g:318-356).

The verb stems have a privileged place in the grammar. The verb stem
is the final syllable in the word. It carries special prominence within the
verb word, by virtue of its phonotactics, which differs from those of the
conjunct morphemes. Recall that this is also the only syllable in the word
where the full set of phonetic contrasts occurs; outside the stem they are
severely reduced. The stem is also semantically prominent, being the main
content morpheme. The nature of verb stem prominence is discussed in
Section 4.5.

2.6.2 The 'Classifiers'

The 'classifiers' are the prefixes to the verb stem, though they are
categorized as conjunct prefixes in the template model, they are included in
the verb domain in the bipartite view. As noted, they are not classifiers in
the generally understood meaning of the term (YM:g117). The reasons for
including them in the Verb domain with the verb stem are syntactic. They
mark transitivity and voice or valence, and thus affect the argument
structure of the verb stem. The system is not entirely productive and the
verb stems are listed with classifiers in the dictionary and appendices. The
combination of a classifier and a verb stems is called a 'verb unit' in
Athabaskan parlance, and is considered an important unit in word formation
in the literature on Athabaskan. Young and Morgan give many examples of
classifier + verb stem combinations, both productive and frozen in their
grammar (g117-127). There are many non-compositional or
conventionalized combinations in the grammar; this aspect of the
morphology is captured by the Athabaskan term 'verb theme' and 'verb
base' (see section 2.7.3). But in both the grammar and the dictionary,
Young and Morgan always provide the reader with the classifier + verb stem
unit.

The classifiers are under prosodic constraints, and they are the source of
a famous series of phonological alternations across Athabaskan. A classifier
does one of three things in the phonology: it is either absorbed by the stem

initial consonant, incorporated into the coda of the Aux stem if that syllable
is open, or it is deleted. It does not appear as a CV on the verb stem. In
effect, affixation to the verb stem is barred (this is discussed further in
Section 3.6.1). In (21) and (22) are forms with the *ł*-classifier in the 1st and
2nd singular forms of the ø-imperfective of *yisdzid* 'I shake it in a pan'. The
2nd singular *ni* (22) is an open syllable, and the classifier *ł-* surfaces in the
coda of this syllable. It has deleted in (21), when the Aux stem is *(y)ish;*
there is no legitimate position for it. In (23) and (24), the classifier has
deleted but it has spread its value for voicing [-voi], to the stem initial
fricative, which appears in its voiceless reflex (see Chapter 5). In (25) the d-
classifier is present.

(21) yis dzid
      [(y)ish   ] [ł   dzid   ]
      [øimp/1s] ['cl' 'agitate, shake':imp]
      [Aux   ] [Verb   ]
      'I shake it in a pan' (YM:d774)

(22) nił dzid
      [ni   ] [ł   dzid   ]
      [øimp/2s] ['cl' 'agitate, shake':imp]
      [Aux   ] [Verb   ]
      'you shake it in a pan'

(23) yis sééh
      [(y)ish   ] [ł   zééh (=sééh)]
      [øimp/1s] ['cl' 'cure'   ]
      [Aux   ] [Verb   ]
      'I make it pliant, cure it' (YM:d776)

(24) ni sééh
      [ni   ] [ł   zééh (=sééh)]
      [øimp/2s] ['cl' 'cure'   ]
      [Aux   ] [Verb   ]
      'you make it pliant'

(25) yi dlóós
      [yi   ] [d   lóós   ]
      [øimp/3s] ['cl' 'lead (animate object)']
      [Aux   ] [Verb   ]
      'it's being lead' (YM:g120)

The effect of the *d*-classifier on the initial consonants of the stem is
called the 'd-effect'; there is an extensive literature on the subject. The full
set of classifier alternations have been discussed in YM, Kari (1976),

McDonough (1990) and (2001). An overview of classifier phonology will be given in Chapter 3.6.1.

What is important to us here is that the classifier is a prefix on the stem and belongs with the stem in the domain Verb. It has its own phonology, arguably a result of the constraints on the verb stem which prevent material coming between the stem boundary and the domain boundary. As a result, the classifier is forced to either incorporate into the stem of the preceding syllable, or delete. In any case its presence may be seen by its phonological effect on the stem-initial consonant.

2.7   ATHABASKAN TERMINOLOGY

Table 8 is a reference table that provides a list of commonly used Athabaskan terms and their definitions. I will adhere to the terminology used in the literature on the Athabaskan languages as much as possible, to avoid the confusion of introducing new terms and to facilitate reference to any discussion of the terms elsewhere.

2.7.1   Null Morphemes

Positions VII, VIII and IX in the template contain empty or null morphemes, marked with ø in Young and Morgan and many other Athabaskan grammars. These positions are obligatory in the verb. They carry all the obligatory morphosyntactic specification necessary in a fully inflected verb. The null morphemes are used in the position classes to represent this specification when it is not associated to a sound form. Generally speaking (not exclusively, see the morpheme list), there are null morphemes for the Mode, for the canonical imperfective (ø-imperfective), for the 3rd person subject position, and for the default classifier prefix. (26) shows a verb with a ø classifier and an Aux stem in the 3rd singular ø imperfective, -i. This verb form also has a disjunct prefix, na- 'downward'. The glosses demonstrate the assumptions of the bipartite model about the role of the Aux stem. In this view the Aux stem is always present, as one of the two obligatory parts of the verb; therefore any default specification is at the stem-level in the grammar, not at the word-level. We'll return to this point in the next section.

(26)   naa baas
        na   # [(i)   ] [ø   baas   ]
        'downward' # [øimp/3s] ['cl' 'hooplike or circular object':imp]
             D   # [Aux] [Verb   ]
        'It (a hooplike or circular object) rolls downward' (YM:g319)

Table 8 A reference table of basic Athabaskan terminology.

Verb complex	A grammatical word a fully inflected form, constituting a proposition. The verb word.
Verb stem	Rightmost morpheme in the complex, monosyllabic, a 'content' morpheme, prominent in the word on several levels.
'Classifiers'	Misnamed prefixes to *Verb stem* a kind of valence or voice marker. YM:g117
Verb unit	The *Classifier + Verb stem*
Verb theme	The *Classifier + Verb stem* 'plus any thematic prefixes' YM:g117 *Verb unit* + supplementary material from the conjunct and disjunct domains which may constitute a particular meaning unit, often used with non-transparent meaning concatenations.
Mode	The name for the conjugational markers of Pos VII, Athabaskan's "tense", primarily concerned with telicity (perfective/ imperfectives). Obligatory w/ subject marking
Qualifiers	A set of Pos VI conjunct prefixes, little studied. Called 'aspectual' prefixes by YM who observe they are an 'ancient stratum in the language'. '*Qualifier*' is Kari's term (1990), probably basically subaspectaul, contributing to event semantics.
'Deictic subject'	Agreement markers of Pos IV that bind subject arguments.
Disjunct	The leftmost domain in the verb, a proclitic domain.
Conjunct	The middle or Aux domain, the second syntactic entity in the verb, containing obligatory subject and mode marking (see the *Base Paradigms*.
Base Paradigms	The term YM use for their paradigm sets of inflected *Mode* conjugations (mode/subject agreement) that are the base of the conjunct or Aux domain.
D-effect	Mutations on the initial consonants of the *Verb stem* caused by the adjacency of the segment /d/, which does not surface outside the onset of the stem.

This form is glossed with a null classifier. The specification for the 3rd person ø-imperfective is the default *i*, (the vowel quality of the default vowel in (26) is contextual). In the template, these positions contain null morphemes for 3rd person and ø-imperfective. In the Base Paradigms these are not null. Another way of saying this is that any default values for phonological specification are given at the stem level; that is to say, all verb words have an Aux stem and all Aux stems have a phonological specification, though it may be the default *(y)i* (the onset glide is epenthetic, a response to word onset constraints). The surface form of the vowel is the default specification –*i*, based on the phonological constraints in the language. The account of the Aux stem in the model also relates to the term 'pepet vowel' and 'peg element'.

2.7.2   The 'Peg' Elements and the Aux Base

The Athabaskan term 'peg elements' (or 'pepet vowel' in Sapir's usage (Young and Morgan do not use this term)) refers to the process of filling out the verb to its minimal two syllable form because of the presence of null morphemes. In (27), all the essential morphemes except the verb stem are default; that is the Aux stem (øimp/3rd) and the classifier (ø).

(27)   yi tsid
     [(y)i   ] [ø   tsid   ]
     [øimp/3s] ['cl' 'pound, beat(plural objects)':imp]
     [Aux   ] [Verb   ]
     's/he pounds it' (YM:d777)

In the Young and Morgan paradigms for this form (d775, g201), the ø-imperfective 3rd singular form is listed as *yi-*. A version of this morpheme gloss that is imposed rigid adherence to the template, where the Mode and subject are separate morphemes, in separate positions, would be as in (28).

(28)   yi tsid
     [ø   ø   ] [ø   tsid   ]
     [Mode subject] ['cl' 'pound, beat(plural objects)':imp]
     [VII   VIII] [IX X   ]
     [Aux   ] [Verb   ]
     's/he pounds it' (YM:d777)

This gloss would require the addition of a 'peg element' *yi* to stand in for the null elements, necessary because of the bisyllabic minimality requirements. In this view, the minimality is stipulated. But the 'peg element' analysis ignores the fact that there is specific morphosyntactic specification for the null elements; they are associated to conjugations. The Young and Morgan approach, using the conjugations of the Base Paradigms as the foundation for the prefix complex, acknowledges the paradigmatic nature of this variation. They list *yi* in the 3rd singular cell of the ø imperfective paradigm.

In the bipartite view adopted, the notion 'peg element' is not necessary because the structure of the verb requires an Aux as one of the two elements in the compound that makes up a verb. As a result an Aux stem is always present in the verb, though it itself may carry default specification. The word is minimally two syllables long because of its morphological structure, not through stipulation. The *yi*, if it is default, fills out the cell in the 3rd singular form of the ø-imperfective paradigm. Thus we get the canonical form in example (27): the *yi* is the Aux stem, the 3rd singular of the ø - imperfective conjugation.

Morphemes from the Qualifier and Agr group, or the disjunct prefixes (as in 2.4) may be affixed to the Aux stem. In fact an argument can be put forth that the Extended Paradigm parts of YM's Base and Extended Paradigms are compositional, they simply a AGR prefix attached to a 3rd default form of the conjugation (AGR $j = i \rightarrow ji$). Insofar as they are compositional, they don't need to be included in the conjugation sets.

Thus in the bipartite view, we assume that there is a default specification in the Aux stem in every verbal form. This assumption will be of particular relevance to a discussion of phonological alternations of vowel length and quality over the disjunct/conjunct boundary, and in the discussion of epenthesis in the next chapter.

2.7.3   The 'Verb Theme' and 'Verb Base'

The terms 'verb base' and 'verb theme' are used in Athabaskan to indicate groups of morphemes within the verb complex. They refer to ways in which meaning units are constructed from the verbal morphemes and to the distinctions between functional, derivational (adverbials) and 'thematic' prefixes. Importantly, these terms encompass both compositional and non-compositional groupings, as well as morphosyntactic processes, though the terms themselves are not defined cearly and can be a source of confusion.

YM (g117) define a verb theme as "the basic units composed of stem + classifier + thematic prefix, if any". This is demonstrated in (29) and (30), where the verb theme is the classifier + stem combination, $ø'\acute{a}$, meaning to 'move/handle a single round object'. I have given glosses to the forms YM provide; the pages for the paradigm charts and listings the glosses are based on are (d407) and (d427) respectively.

(29)   ha'íí '$\acute{a}$
    ha   # ['(a) (h)i (y)ish   ] [ø   '$\acute{a}$]
    'up' # [3i   ser øimp/1s] ['cl' 'handle a single round object':imp]
    D   # [Aux   ] [Verb   ]
    the sun came up'

(30)   háá '$\acute{a}$
    ha   ná # [(i)   ] [ø   '$\acute{a}$]
    'up' rev # [øimp/3s] ['cl' 'handle a single round object':imp]
    D   # [Aux   ] [Verb   ]
    'I took it out'

The term 'thematic' is often used to refer to the non-compositionality or opaqueness of morpheme combinations in the verb complex. This reflects the fact that many morpheme combinations are lexicalized or have conventionalized meanings. 'Thematic' morphemes may include grammatical prefixes, such as the 3i object agreement marker '*(a)*, which YM provide as part of a theme in a number of forms. In (31) and (32) are example of two uses of this morpheme, provided by YM, which exhibit this distinction between productivity and opaqueness (g39). The form in (31) is compositional, in (32) it is 'thematic' by their definition.

(31)   'as há
        ['(a) (y)ish   ] [ø   á   ]
        [3i   øimp/1s] ['cl' 'eat']
        [Aux   ] [Verb   ]
        'I'm eating (something)'

(32)   'ash zhish
        ['(a) (y)ish   ] [l   zhish   ]
        [3i   øimp/1s] ['cl' 'move in a rhythmic manner']
        [Aux   ] [Verb   ]
        'I'm dancing'

However, a case can be made that the form in (32) reflects a verb-internal morphosyntactic process in the same way as the one in (a); 'I'm moving (something) in a rhythmic manner'. The 3i marker "something" binds an argument of the verb from having verb external reference. Evidence for this is the presence of the d-classifier (d + ł → l) in the verb domain. The *d*-classifier is characteristic of constructions such as the passive, medio-passive, reflexives and reciprocals (g117), where an argument of the verb is bound within the complex, here, arguably by the existential quantifier 3i 'something'. A discussion of the morphosyntactic processes that occur within the verb is beyond the scope of the present work. I offer this here to indicate that that the term 'verb theme' is a general descriptive term, not a technical one.

For instance, YM write "There is no apparent relationship between ł-classifier in its transitivizing and in its thematic role in themes such as: di--łhił..." (g119), again associating the term 'thematic' with non-compositional meaning. The term 'verb theme' is used more broadly to mean lexicalized combinations of morphemes that include the classifier + stem (Verb) base. In the form *di--łhił* 'be dark, colored', for instance, the prefix *d(i)* (pos VIb) combines with the classifier + stem (Verb) combination *łhił*: [d(i) − *stem*]$_{AUX}$ [łhił]$_{VERB}$. This unit can be conjugated, by using the Base Paradigms: [d(i) − *ish*]$_{AUX}$ [łhił]$_{VERB}$, 'I'm tanned.' Notions like 'verb theme' are important because they address non-compositionality of the morpheme concatenations, which is an important aspect of the productivity of the morphology. There is extensive homophony among the (pos VI) Qu prefixes; the *di-* Qu morpheme for instance, is also a component of several other meanings, such as the inceptive aspect (as in (9)). In fact, YM (g38) lists 14 different meanings for the morpheme *d(i)-*.

The term 'verb base' is a more ambiguous term, and it is not clearly defined in the grammar. It partially overlaps in meaning with the term 'verb theme' in that it refers to the classifier + stem and particular prefixes. YM provides long lists of verb bases in their discussion of the morphemes, and the verb base often determines how a verb is conjugated. I refer the reader to the discussion on the morphemes in the template (YM:g39-127), which include many examples and discussions of the behavior of verb bases. In this study I have avoided the use of these terms, I use the term 'verb unit', as in basic verb unit, to indicate the classifier + verb stem conbination that comprises the category Verb in the word.

Both these terms refer to important and open questions relating to the nature of the lexicon in Athabaskan; what kinds of information do language learners store? How are these forms stored and accessed? What is the working distinction between function and content morphemes in a polysynthetic language? What are the grammatical constraints on morphological productivity? These questions are not only important to Navajo and Athabaskan, but to broader issues in linguistic theory, language acquisition and language processing. They have the potential of expanding our ideas about the nature of the lexicon because they represent a very different language type from the kinds that formal theories were constructed to explain. A good working model of the verbal structure and a solid description of the sound profile are necessary to investigate of these phenomena.

2.8   SUMMARY

A model of the structure of the verb has been presented in this chapter as a basis for word formation and a study of the phonological and phonetic properties of Navajo speech. In this model, called the bipartite model, the verb word is not a single constituent, it's a compound of two separable parts. Two domains, an Aux and a Verb, each comprised of a inflected stem, are joined to produce the core verb. Prefixes may attach to these stems within their domains. The Verb domain is the combination of a classifier and a verb stem (*łbą́ą́s* 'move a hooplike object'). The Aux domain has, as its stem, a form from the conjugational Base Paradigms of YM (g200-01); these forms indicate particular conjugational modes inflected for person and number (*(y)ish*, øimp/1st). These two entities, the Aux and Verb stems, are the foundation of word formation in Navajo. Compounded, they comprise a fully inflected verb, but they are distinct entities and the boundary between them is an obvious boundary in the speech signal. Within the Aux, two kinds of prefixes are found: a set of qualifier prefixes (pos VI) and a set of agreement markers (VI and V). Finally, morphemes from the disjunct domain (labeled 'proclitics') may attach to the left edge of this compound. A schema of this structure is represented in (33).

(33)   [Proclitics # [AGR [af – stem]]$_{Aux}$ [af - stem]$_{Verb}$]$_{Verb\ Word}$
     D   # [Aux   ]   [Verb   ]

The diagram in (34) captures the reassignments of the template positions to the bipartite structure. There are three majors points of reassignment: a major break between the final and penult syllable marking the compound boundary, the affiliation of the classifier prefix to the Verb as part of the verb unit, and the merging of the pos VII and VII morphemes into inflectional paradigms, which are assigned to the morphological category stem. The underlined elements represent the two stems:

(34)   0-III # [IV/V- VI(a,b,c)- <u>VII/VIII</u>] [IX <u>Verb stem</u>]
     D # [Aux   ] [Verb   ]

The glosses throughout the book are presented in the bipartite structure, but morpheme references to the positions in the template are given so as to facilitate cross-reference to both a template version of the morphology, and to appropriate sections in the YM gammars. The bipartite model is intended to represent a native speaker's working knowledge of the structure of the verbal complex. It is designed to support morphosyntactic processes and to capture morphophonemic alternations in a maximally transparent way. In the remainder of the book we will examine the phonological and phonetic properties of the elements in the verb.

---

[1] The parenthesis in the glosses indicate alternations that very often have a simple phonological basis, such as indicating the epenthetic glide that appears in word initial position ((y)ish-cha → yishcha) due to a constraint on syllables having onsets, etc.

[2] I use Kari's term Qualifiers here instead of 'aspectual', the term that Young and Morgan use, to distinguish them from the Mode morphemes, which are also aspectual. See Sussman (2002) and Hargus (2000). The term 'classifier' is a misnomer, these are valence or voice markers (Axelord 1999). This term is the source of much confusion. I'll assume this name and use quotes with this term throughout the text.

[3] Young and Morgan capitalize the verb stems and list them by their imperfective forms in Appendix V, the appendix that lists the stems sets for the verb stems. These stem sets are the second of the two major paradigms in the verb. (The first is the Base Paradigms, see discussion.) When referring to the verb, I'll follow the YM convention and capitalize these forms, presenting them as they are entered in the Root/Stem/Theme dictionary of Appendix V.

[4] The transitional marker yi- is glossed as (y)i. The claim is that this prefix is a vowel. The reasons are due to the alternations it effects on the following vowel, making it long. It surfaces as yi- when it is in a position to need an onset, i.e. at the edge of a domain. Therefore the y is epenthetic. For more complete discussion see the paradigms in Young and Morgan 1987 where it appears, McDonough 1990, and chapter 6 on the phonology.

---

⁵ Examples such as these may be found in the grammar by using Appendix I (YM:g202ff). This appendix lists the fully elaborated paradigms, consisting of the possible combinations of the Base conjugations plus the combinations of disjunct and conjunct prefixes. At the bottom of each paradigm column are listed examples of the forms from that paradigm. See Chapter 6 for further discussion on using the Young and Morgan grammar.

⁶ The classifier prefix is under special prosodic constraints (Chapter 3.6.1). If the Aux stem is an open syllable, the classifier can move into its coda position, otherwise it deletes. The claim of the bipartite model is that appearing in the coda of the Aux stem does not affect its affiliation to the Verb stem domain.

Chapter 3

PHONOLOGY

3.0 INTRODUCTION

This chapter provides a basic outline of the phonology of the Navajo language. My goal is to give a descriptive account of the major principled phonological processes in the language, and this will serve as a basis of an investigation of its phonetic structure.

Some alternation patterns are complex enough to require separate studies in themselves, such as the consonant harmony system, the classifier effects, and the alternations of the stems. Examinations of these alternation patterns in the past have been based on orthographic evidence and have been limited by a lack of explicit knowledge of the language's phonetic structure, which this book begins to address. I will give an overview of these processes in this chapter.

We will assume the morphological structure of the verb shown in (1), as discussed in Chapter 2, as a base for the phonology. To review, there are three domains in the verb, the disjunct (D), the conjunct or auxiliary (Aux), and the verb stem (Verb). The basic verb is a syntactic compound: the compounded entities are the final two domains, Aux and Verb, where each domain has a stem as a base. The Aux stem is equivalent to the conjugations of the Base Paradigms (YM:g200-1). The prefixes to the verb stem are the classifiers. The prefixes in the Aux domain attach to the Aux stem: the Agreement (Agr) markers of Pos. IV (direct object) and V ('deictic subject') and the Qualifiers (Qu) morphemes of Pos. VI. The disjunct morphemes are clitics.

(1)   [Clitics # [Agr [Qu – stem]$_{Aux}$ ['cl' - stem]$_{Verb}$]$_{Verb\ Word}$
        D   # [Aux   ]   [Verb   ]

The minimal verb consists of an Aux stem and a Verb stem. We will refer to any disjunct and conjunct (or Aux) morpheme groupings to the left of the verb stem as the 'prefix complex' when we want to discuss them as an entirety. This is not a formal term, but I use it as a rhetorical convenience, since this marks a major division in the word, and is an acknowledgment of the paradigmatic variation that occurs with many of the morpheme

41

combinations which precede the verb stem. Many of these concatenations are captured as paradigms in YM's Appendix I, *The Model Paradigms*, in which they use, as a foundation for affixation, the conjugations of the Base Paradigms (the Aux stems). This insight is captured by the model in (1). Thus I will refer here for convenience to the divisions in the verb word as a 'prefix complex' plus a 'verb stem', but the model in (1) underlies these terms.

3.1   PHONOTACTICS

The three domains of the verb are marked by phonotactic differences. Table 1, repeated here as Table 9, lists the phonemes from Young and Morgan (for their IPA transcriptions see Chapter 1). There are two focal characteristics of the phonemic contrasts: the inventory is primarily coronal, and it can be divided into two main groups dependent on their alternation patterns: the stops and the fricatives.

Table 9 Navajo consonants in the orthography of Young and Morgan 1987.

p	t, d, t'				k, g, k'	kw, gw	'
		ts, dz, ts'	ch, j, ch'				
		tl, dl, tl'					
	s, z		sh, zh		x, gh		h
	ł, l						
m	n						
w			y				

The coronal-heavy inventory means that the phonemic contrasts are predominantly constructed with features other than place of articulation, mainly manner and laryngeal contrasts. Bilabials are rare and they have a limited distribution, occurring only in word initial (*b*) or stem initial (*b* and *m*) position. The stops (except the labials) exhibit a three-way laryngeal contrast: plain (unaspirated), aspirated and ejective (or glottalized). The stops also have three different kinds of releases that correspond to the three fricative types in the inventory: plain, fricative and lateral. The stops are stable; they do not show phonological alternations.

The second group of phonemes are the fricative group; this group includes the glides and nasals. There are two sets of central strident fricatives and one set of lateral fricatives: the alveolar, *s, z* [s, z], the alveolo-palatal *sh, zh* [ʃ, ʒ], and the lateral ł, l [ɬ l]. The velar fricatives, *x, gh* [x ɣ], exhibit considerable contextual variation, and they tend to lenite to approximants, which are expressed as glides in the orthography (Chapter 5.3). 'True' glides occur only in a small number of lexical items; generally the glides that appear are either epenthetic –as consonantal versions of the following vowel– or they are contextual alternants of the coronal and back fricatives. We will examine the coronal and dorsal glides in Section 3.4 on glide alternations. The *h* symbol represents both a velar fricative and a syllable-final glottal fricative, depending on its position in the syllable (onset versus coda) (YM:xiv).

The distribution of the phonemic inventory is strictly constrained The single place in the lexicon where the full set of the consonantal contrasts are found is in the onset of the verb and noun stems. Outside this position, these contrasts are severely reduced. For example, Table 10 is a list of the contrasts in the conjunct, or auxiliary domain, taken from the morpheme charts of YM (g37-38). Manner, laryngeal and most of the place contrasts are neutralized in the conjunct domain. This distribution constraint is a determining characteristic of the sound profile of the language, and it is important to keep it in mind in a discussion of the phonology[1].

Table 10 Consonantal contrasts in conjunct (Aux) domain (Navajo orthography)

	bilabial	alveolar	alveolo-palatal	back	glottal
stops	b	d			'
fricatives		s, z	sh, zh	h	
nasals		n			
lateral fricatives		ł,l			

The vowel contrasts follow this same pattern. There are four principle vowel qualities: two front vowels, *i* and *e*, a round vowel, *o,* and a low vowel, *a* (see Chapter 5). There are length, nasality and tone contrasts in the vowel system, but these contrasts are only found in the nucleus of the stem (see Chapter 1 for discussion of the vowel contrasts). There are no nasal or long vowel contrasts in the conjunct domain. The disjunct domain contains a set of morphemes with stem-like phonotactic properties (the 'postpositinal stems'), but outside this group the contrasts are similar to those found in the conjunct domain. Thus the contrasts in Table 9 are not robust outside the stem. Tonal contrasts are also reduced outside the stem morphemes, with low tone as the default tone, as YM notes (xiii) (see the discussion in McDonough 1999).

Kari (1976) and YM also note that, in the conjunct domain, the default vowel is the high front vowel *i*, and many instances of non-default vowels are phonological variants of it. The low vowel *a* associated with the laryngeal consonants *h* and ', and *o* with labialization in the *ho, hwi* alternation. In Section 3.2.1 the epenthetic status of the conjunct vowels will be discussed. There is a greater range of vowel contrasts, including tone, among the paradigms of the Aux stem (Base Paradigms). The vowel features are often associated to specific conjugations, such as the *ó* in the optative conjugation or the high tone associated with the perfective (Kari 1976), as such have a grammatical rather than contrastive function.

The disjunct domain has a wider range of contrasts than the conjunct; there are ejectives among these morphemes for instance, as well as vowel contrasts not present in the conjunct domain (such as quality, tone, length contrasts), and these morphemes also may have codas (g37); (2) demonstrates a variety of these phenomena; the first five are postpositional stems (pos Ib), the final one is the reversionary (Id) or iterative marker (pos II).

(2)   ch'í-:   out horizontally
       ch'aa-:   travel, visit, away from home base
       k'e-:   loosen, undo, take down
       k'é-:   peace, friendliness, good human relations
       tsíts'á-:   away from the fire or water
       ná-   reversionary / iterative

Most of these contrasts are confined to a single disjunct position, Ib, a position termed Adverbial-Thematic. YM notes that many of these position Ib morphemes "...are postpositional stems that have found their way into the prefix complex as bound morphemes..."[2] (g42). 'Postpositional' stems retain some of the phonotactic properties of stems (see YM:g26-36 for discussion of the function and distribution of postpositional stems). This is the position of noun incorporation in the Athabaskan languages that have incorporation (Axelrod).

Outside the stems, the set of contrastive features that occur is almost exclusively coronal, without the rich manner and laryngeal contrasts found in the stem onset. The vowel contrasts are also reduced, and the default vowel is marked as high and front[3]. Because of morpheme ordering and bisyllabicity in the verb, the stem seldom, if, ever, is found in word initial position. Thus the phonemes of the inventory in Table 8 are not in initial position in the word, and their prosodic position does not vary. In fact the phonemic inventory is, in effect, a list of the possible stems onsets.

This distribution pattern is a striking aspect of the phonological profile of the verb word. It means, for one, that the stems are phonotactically quite prominent. We will see in Chapters 4 and 5 when we discuss the phonetic profile of the verb that several factors conspire to make stems prominent in the word. The phonotactic distribution is the most evident among them. These phonotactics and their phonetic realization are part of a systematic and characteristic profile that is reflected in the phonetic and prosodic structure. We can characterize this acoustic profile as one with a prominent syllable at the right edge, preceded by a more compressed group of pre-stem morphemes. There is a distinct break between the stem and the prefix complex. These two groups have quite discrete phonotactics, as we've seen, and, by extension, a discrete phonology and phonetics. The pre-stem complex is comprised of two domains, and we'll see that these domains have distinct phonological and phonetic properties as well as distinct syntactic and semantic ones, although this is a lesser distinction than the one between the pre-stem group and the final syllable of the word.

One consideration is the role this profile plays in the prosodic organization of the word. The data indicates that very little evidence can be construed for organization above the level syllable in the grammar of Navajo at least. Tonal phenomena seem to support this (McDonough 1999, 2002). The question of how the organization and acoustic profile of the word varies across Athabaskan is an interesting one, though unstudied. In this chapter I will review the principle phonological constraints that appear to be active in the grammar, as a basis for a discussion of the phonetics.

3.2   SYLLABLE STRUCTURE

One of the several characteristics that separates stems from affixes is their syllable structure. These two types of morphemes –stems and prefixes– have different syllable structure constraints, as shown in Table 11.

Table 11 Syllable Structure Constraints

Morpheme	Stem	Prefix
Syllable Structure	CVVC	CV

Stem shapes may be checked by examining the roots in the YM Root/ Stem / Theme Index (Appendix V g318-356), the forms of the Base Paradigms (Appendix I g206-250), as well as the list of nouns (g1-8) and the discussion of postpositional stems (g26-35). Otherwise conjunct and disjunct morphemes are almost all CV. In addition, Navajo also has an onset condition, which is apparent in the initial glide alternations in forms like *(y)ish* (øimp/1st) and *(w)oh* (øimp/2[nd]d); the glides appear when these forms are in word-initial position (YM:g113-15).

3.2.1 Epenthesis

Vocalic epenthesis is a more complex phenomenon. McDonough (1996) has shown that the vowels are arguably epenthetic if we assume that the Qu and Agr morphemes are prefixed to the Aux stem. In this view, the prefixes to the Aux stem are non-syllabic consonants; a syllable driven fix-up process occurs when the concatenation of a prefix to a base produces an illegal consonant sequence, (e.g. CC). The prefixes can be seen to exhibit alternations depending on the Aux base they attach to. If the Base Paradigm form is vowel initial (such as the ø imperfective), the prefix appears in the onset of that syllable, as in (3). If the Base paradigm is consonant initial, the prefix appears as a separate syllable with the default vowel *i-*, as in (4). The forms in both (3) and (4) have as a Qu (pos. VI) prefix, *d-³* 'open' (d310), with 1ˢᵗ person form of the n-imperfective and ø-imperfective conjugations, *nish* and *(y)ish* respectively (g200). When *d-* is prefixed to the øimp/1ˢᵗ stem *-ish* it appears in onset, as *dish-*, but when it is prefixed to the *-nish*, the result is *dinish*, as the concatenation otherwise would result in the illegal sequence **dnish*. Note that if the prefix were *di-* the result in the ø-imperfective would be *diish*.

(3)   d - ish → dish-   (*diish-)
       dish gééd (I)
       [d   ish   ] [ø   gééd]
       ['open' øimp/1ˢᵗ] ['cl' 'dig']
       [Aux ·   ] [Verb   ]
       'dig a drain trench, drain it' (YM:d335)

(4)   d- nish → dinish- (*dnish-)
       'ąą dinish tįįh (I)
       'ąą [d   nish   ] [ø   tįįh   ]
       'there' ['open' nimp/1ˢᵗ] ['cl' 'handle (a SSO)']
              [Aux   ] [Verb   ]
       'to open it (a door)' (YM:d327)

(5) is another example of the epenthesis process, shown occuring with a vocalic prefix, the semelfactive (y)i-, which surfaces as a vowel (g104). This form raises the issue of long vowels in the conjunct domain. The long vowel in this form is derived from the concatenation of two morphemes. The prolongative is a composite of two Qu prefixes, *d-* + *n-*, plus the *i-*semelfactive, to the ø –imperfective/1ˢᵗ form *(y)ish* in (5). Note that the epenthetic account also obviates the need for a rule that deletes the vowel in (3) (**diish*) and allows it in (5).

(5)   d+n+i+ish → diniish-
       diniish jih (I)
       [d   n   i   ish   ] [ø   gééd]
       [prolongative semelfactive øimp/1ˢᵗ] ['cl' 'grab']
       [Aux   ] [Verb   ]
       'to grab it and hang on' (YM:d330)

Many examples of other prefix concatenations of this type can be found throughout the paradigms in the dictionary. These concatenations and alternation patterns make phonological sense if the concatenation is to a base (i.e. to the forms of the conjugational Base Paradigms), and the prefixes are non-syllabic consonants. Insofar as this is the case, then the prefixes in the conjunct domain are non-syllabic, and inflectional. With few exceptions (Pos. Ib in particular) this is also true of the morphemes of the disjunct domain. The nature of theses prefixes comes into play when we examine the durational properties of these domains in the next chapter.

The quality of the prefix vowel *i* in the conjunct domain will be discussed in Section 5.1.5 on the spectral analyses of conjunct vowels.

3.2.2 Stem Alternations

The roots in Navajo are an abstraction over the stems sets, which are sets of aspectually related morphemes (Chapter 2.6.1). An example of a stem set for the verb theme 'chop, cut with an axe' follows, taken at random from Appendix V, the Root / Stem / Theme Index (g318-356). Note the differences over the set in vowel quality and length and in the final consonant. The root is in SMALL CAPS.

(6)   -TSEEŁ: to chop, cut with an axe
        *øtseeł (I), øtsi' (R), *øtsééł (P), *øtsił (F), *øtseeł (O)

The variations among these stems are somewhat systematic, though it is apparently not a fully productive system. The best study of the stem alternations is found in Hardy (1969). It is generally believed that the differences in aspectual shapes arose from the incorporation of suffixal material into the stem (Krauss and Leer 1981, Kari 1976). I refer the reader to their discussion of these stem alternations.

3.2.3 Root Constraints

Root constraints is a term that refers to limits on the distribution of segments that occur within an underived word, root or stem. Navajo root constraints are of interest because of their relationship to the language's consonant harmony system, which we will discuss in Section 3.3. The root constraint in Navajo is simply stated: there are no contrasting features for central coronal fricatives within a morphological category root or stem (noun or verb, including the forms of the Base Paradigms (g200-1) and the postpositional stems (g24)).

Recall the large inventory of coronal consonants in the phonemic inventory in Table 9, and recall that this set is constrained to occur only in the onset of the stem. The coda of the stem allows a more reduced set of segment types: the coronal consonants, minus all the manner, laryngeal and place contrasts (*s, z, sh, zh, ł, n*). Since stems have codas, it is thus possible for a root/stem to have a coronal fricative in both the onset and coda. However, there are constraints on the combinations of consonants that actually occur: they may not have opposing values for anteriority. The following discussion is taken from McDonough (1990).

To frame the constraint we will use the feature [anterior] to capture the distinction between the alveolar and alveolo-palatal fricatives *s, z* [s z] and *sh, zh* [ʃ, ʒ]. The feature [anterior] distinguishes contrasts among coronal consonants more generally, as can be seen in (7).

(7)   s, z, ts, dz   [+anterior, coronal]
      [s, z, tsʰ, ts]
      sh, zh, ch, j   [−anterior, coronal]
      [ʃ, ʒ, tʃʰ, tʃ]

This contrast is a common one, and the feature [anterior] is descriptively valid, so the contrast can be formalized in any theoretical framework.

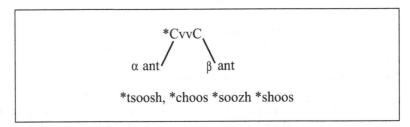

Figure 4 Non-occurring root/stem syllable structures in Navajo.

The root constraint on Navajo disallows opposing values for anteriority within a root/stem. That is to say, roots of the type in Figure 4 do not occur in the language. This is a constraint on the coronal fricatives (*s, z, sh, zh*) and the stops with fricative releases (the *ts* and *ch* series in Table 9). Thus all roots and stems in the lexicon that have two coronal fricatives gestures must share the value for anteriority, as in the examples in (8).

(8)   TSQQS   'to wrinkle, become rugose.'   (g348)
      CH'IISH   'to grate, rasp, file...'   (g322)
      JĮISH   'to smash, crush squeeze...'   (g331)

Note that the lateral fricatives (*l ł*) and laterally released affricates (*tł* series) may appear with both [+anterior] or [− anterior] fricatives within a root/stem, as seen in (9). Thus they do not participate in the constraint.

(9)   LÓÓS   'to lead (one animate object)'   (g337)
      CH'ÍÍŁ   'to strike (lightning)'   (g322)
      LÍÍSH   to leak, spew out...'   (g337)

This constraint extends beyond the stem into the word formation process, resulting in consonantal alternations, i.e. consonant harmony, when two morphemes with opposing values are concatenated. The stem morpheme is the trigger, and the harmony is regressive.

3.3   CONSONANT HARMONY

The consonant harmony system in Athabaskan is an interesting system for several reasons. The first reason relates to the phenomenon of consonant harmony in general. Consonant harmony processes are phonological processes affecting the feature specification of non-adjacent consonants. Consonantal harmony is not common cross-linguistically and when it does occur the generalization is that the process is constrained to harmony among independent articulators. These are the velum (nasal harmony) or (larynx) laryngeal harmony, and the harmony of coronal features. Coronal harmony occurs across Athabaskan. In Navajo, the consonant harmony constraint is identical to the root/stem constraint on the feature [anterior], except that it is carried into the word formation processes.

A second point of interest lies in the function of place of articulation as a principle contrast in phonemic systems. The IPA for instance is organized along one primary dimension according to place of articulation. Most phonological theories are based on a feature system which is predominantly articulatorily defined, making the bias of the system towards place of articulation contrasts. In this sense, the phonemic system in Athabaskan is exceptional; it is a coronal-heavy inventory. The non-coronal places of articulation are velars and bilabials, but bilabial is not a functional contrast, and the velar contrast in fricatives is being lost, conditioned by a lenition process that results in a glide as its vocalic reflex (see Section 3.4). So why would a language with an already reduced set of place of articulation contrasts further reduce its phonemic inventory by disallowing contrasts among the coronal consonants? This question is related to our concerns about the function of contrasts in languages like the Athabaskan languages where the distribution of contrasts is so severely constrained that the notion 'minimal pair' plays little role in determining the phonemic contrasts.

A third point of interest is the domain of the harmony process. It certainly extends to the consonants immediately adjacent to the stem, but it seems to weaken as it moves away into the outer (left) morphemes.

A fourth, related, point is the articulation of the consonants of the contrast. Is this a purely phonological alternation in which the coronal consonants have been outright replaced by a harmonized reflex, or is it a more phonetically based and defined alternation in which there is a more gradient effect? Does it exist within a morphologically defined domain? Other questions involve issues surrounding the differences between dialects of Navajo, in the scope of the harmony process within the utterance, and the

Navajo system's relationship to the broader Athabaskan harmony processes, such as Tahltan's three-way harmony (Shaw 1990).

In this section I will provide a brief description of the harmony process in Navajo. A full examination of this process is beyond what than we can accomplish in this study; instead, the goal of this section is to provide a general phonological description of the harmony alternations, and to provide clearly defined questions concerning the process in Navajo.

3.3.1 Harmony in the Aux Domain

As we saw above in Figure 4, the grammar has a constraint on opposing values of anteriority within roots / stems. We will call this the consonant harmony constraint, given in (10).

(10) * [α ant β ant]$_X$

As a root constraint, it governs the distribution of consonants within the root, and 'X' in (10) is the morphological category root/stem. The harmony process extends this root constraint into the domain of word formation. In (11) is an example of a verb with the Aux stem in the familiar ø imperfective/1st *(y)ish*. In (12) the Aux stem is also *-ish*, but it surfaces as -*is*, because the verb stem is [+ant] *dzį́į́s*, and consonant harmony applies.

(11)   yish ch'id
        [(y)ish   ] [ø   ch'id   ]
        [øimp/1st] ['cl' 'scratch']
        [Aux   ] [Verb   ]
        'to scratch it' (YM:d780)

(12)   yis dzį́į́s
        [(y)ish   ] [ø   dzį́į́s   ]
        [øimp/1st] ['cl' 'pull, tow']
        [Aux   ] [Verb   ]
        'to drag it' (YM:d775)

That the harmony is regressive, from the stem to the prefix groups, is further exemplified by the s-perfective/1st auxiliary, which appears as *sis* in the unmarked case (g201) and alternates to *shish-* when it is adjacent to a [-ant] stem *jool*. (13) and (14) show this alternation, the opposite of that in (11) and (12). Thus, we have examples of an alternation between *sh* and *s* in both directions, dependent on the anteriority of the stem.

(13)   sis tin
      [sis   ] [d   tin   ]
      [sperf/1st] ['cl' stem]
      [Aux   ] [Verb   ]
      'be frozen' (YM:g233,column77)

(14)   shish jool
      [sis   ] [l   jool   ]
      [sperf/1st] ['cl' stem]
      [Aux   ] [Verb   ]
      'lie huddled, cowering' (YM:g233,column77)

The dictionary and grammar are full of these type alternations. The Base Paradigms are listed in their neutral forms (the form that appears with non-harmonizing stems). A search through the dictionary tells us that the Base Paradigms are the principle domain of this alternation; all the forms from the Base Paradigms harmonize to the stems to their right. We can characterize this informally as a regressive harmony rule, spreading the feature for anteriority leftward, as shown in Figure 5.

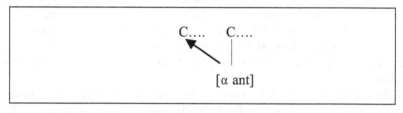

Figure 5 Regressive Consonant Harmony

This regressive harmony from the verb stem to the Aux stem is the basic pattern. Beyond the conjugational forms of the Aux stem however, the consonant harmony process becomes murkier. Recall that the morphemes that are prefixes to Aux stem are the Qualifiers (Pos. VIa, b,c) and the Agreement markers (pos. IV V). These morphemes show alternation patterns that are less straightforward, indicating that outside the Aux stem there are several factors that influence harmony. These factors are not well understood and require special study.

For instance, harmony holds for the 1st person Agr marker *sh-*. This Agr prefix *sh-* harmonizes to *s-*, a process triggered by an Aux in (15) and a verb stem in (16).

(15)   siz taɬ
      [sh   iz   ] [ø   taɬ   ]
      [1st O sperf/3] ['cl' 'act with the feet']
      [Aux   ] [Verb   ]
      'it gave me a kick' (YM:g65)

(16)   soo sił
      [sh   ooh   ] [ł   ził   ]
      [1st O sperf/2nd] ['cl' 'grab']
      [Aux   ] [Verb   ]
      'you two are grabbing me' (YM:g65)

One the other hand, the Agr marker *j*- from Pos V 'deictic subject', undergoes harmony, but it is optional in many cases. YM gives the forms in (17). This morpheme has a special status in the grammar; it appears to resist epenthesis and tends to metathesize into a coda, surfacing in several alternate forms, as discussed in Section 3.7.

(17) dziz diz ~ jiz diz   'she spun it' (YMg77) (optional)

In addition, although there are coronal fricatives among the Qualifier prefixes of Pos VI, the harmony data on these is not straightforward. In large part this is because the alternations themselves are not well understood (g64-66). YM reports alternations between glides and fricatives among these morphemes. Although this is a pattern we are familiar with from the stem alternation (in Section 3.2.2), the nature of the alternation pattern in these Qu prefixes is less well understood and less obviously phonological in nature. It will be important to understand the systematicty of these alternations before we can determine the extent to which they are targets for harmony.

There are further constraints on the harmony process. For instance, harmony apparently does not affect the disjunct prefixes. YM reports forms such as (18) throughout the grammar, where the disjunct prefix *ch'í* (Ib) does not harmonize to the stem *ts'óód*, even though the regressive harmony changes the value for the nimp/1st *nish* [-ant] to *nis* [+ant] to match the stem's [+ant] value.

We also found this to be the case in our data. Although the disjunct prefixes have a 1st person indirect object morpheme *sh-* (disjunct: Pos Ia (g42)), YM does not list an alternate anterior form (*s-*) for this morpheme, implying that this morpheme does not undergo harmony. As such, the morphemes of the disjunct domain are outside the scope of the constraint. This is not surprising, as Sapir and Hoijer (1967), Kari (1976), YM (1980, 1987) and others report the disjunct / conjunct boundary as a domain boundary for the application of morphophonemic rules.

A complete examination of the harmony process in Navajo, and in Athabaskan, requires an independent study, with carefully designed word lists. The study would benefit from including an articulatory study of tongue body shape in order to determine the nature of this alternation. It is clear, however, that a characterization of the harmony process, in Navajo at least, as a fully regressive harmony process triggered by the stem is inaccurate. The harmony is more constrained. The exact nature and scope of this constraint remains to be studied: it may be by domain, or it may be constrained by a morpheme's adjacency to a anterior fricative, or (most likely) a mix of phonological, paradigmatic and morphological factors. It might be influenced by intervening segments, and it could also be the case that dialectic variation is a factor in the scope of the harmony rule. The data indicates only that the Aux stem regularly harmonizes to the verb stem. Beyond that the case is open.

(18)   ch'ínís ts'óód
        ch'í # [nish   ] [ø   ts'óód   ]
        'out' # [nimp/1st] ['cl' 'stretch']
        Ib   # [VII/VIII] [IX   X   ]
        D   # [Aux   ] [Verb   ]
        'I lean out' (YM:d294)

3.4   FRICATIVE AND GLIDE REFLEXES

As noted, the fricative group includes both fricatives and approximants, a grouping which is discussed more thoroughly in Chapter 5. One of the reasons for this grouping is the reflex sets that stem-initial fricatives undergo. I review the facts here (see also McDonough 1990).

The fricatives in the stem-initial position exhibit a set of contextual reflexes. The first reflex is voicing. Despite the phoneme chart in Table 9, voicing is contextual rather than contrastive in fricatives. There are two voiced environments for stem-initial fricatives: intervocalic and immediately following a voiced consonant. The voiceless environment occurs after a voiceless fricative, such as ł and *sh/s*. Recall that the verb stems are listed in their voiced reflex in the Root / Stem / Theme index (appendix V) of YM (g:136-159).

In (19) and (20) are two forms with the verb theme *ølááh* 'to gather', whose verb stem begins with a lateral fricative. In the imperfective conjugation it is preceded by *sh,* the coda of the Base Paradigm's ø-imperfective / 1st singular form *(y)ish*; this voiceless fricative creates a voiceless environment for the stem-initial consonant, so the lateral appears in its voiceless reflex ł in (19). In (20) the Aux stem is CV; the lateral fricative is intervocalic and it surfaces in its voiced reflex *l*.

(19)   náhásh łááh (I)
        ná # [h   (y)ish   ] [ø   łááh   ]
        'up' # [ser. øimp/1st] ['cl' 'gather objects']
        D   # [Aux   ] [Verb   ]
        'I gather them, pick them up' (YM:d531)

(20)   náhá láá' (P)
        ná   # [h   i   ] [ø   láá'   ]
        'up' # [ser. øperf/3rd] ['cl' 'gather objects']
        D   # [Aux   ] [Verb   ]
        'he gathers them, picks them up' (YM:d531)

In (21) and (22), the initial segment of the stem surfaces as a voiceless
fricative *sh*, due to the presence of the *ł*-classifier, a voiceless lateral
fricative. In a typical pattern the *ł*-classifier does not surface – it is deleted –
but not before it has passed on its value for voicing to the stem-initial
fricative. Thus, the initial fricative surfaces as voiceless in both (21) and
(22), despite the surface intervocalic environment of (22). The reflex of the
stem is the single indication of the presence of the lateral classifier *ł*.

(21)   yish shééh (I)
        [(y)ish   ] [ł   zhééh]
        [øimp/1st] ['cl' 'mow']
        [Aux   ] [Verb   ]
        'to mow it (grass hay)' (YM:d789)

(22)   yí shéé' (P)
        [(y)í   ] [ł   zhéé']
        [yperf/1st] ['cl' 'mow']
        [Aux   ] [Verb   ]
        'to mow it (grass hay) (perfective)' (YM:d789)

These are the contexts for the voicing of all stem-initial fricatives. The
phonological voicing contrast among fricatives in Navajo may be best
characterized as a lenition contrast and not voicing, a phenomena that has
also been observed in Northern Athabaskan languages (Holton 2002). I will
continue to refer to this as a phonological 'voicing' contrast for simplicity.
The nature of this contrast is examined in Chapter 5.

There is a third alternation that these fricatives undergo. When they are
adjacent to a *d*-segment (an unaspirated coronal stop) from either the *d*-
classifier or the 1st dual subject marker *–ii(d)*, they exhibit a reflex that is
known as the Athabaskan 'd-effect'. Basically, they absorb the *d*-segment
into the onset of the stem. This alternation is discussed more fully in
Section 3.6.1. The result of the 'd-effect' is an alternation between the
fricative and an affricate reflex. Thus for the three basic fricatives, [+ant]
and [-ant] fricative, *z* and *zh* respectively, and the lateral fricative *l* (in
keeping with the YM convention of using the voiced reflex as basic), each
surfaces as one of three reflexes, depending on context, giving us the
fricative reflex sets shown in Table 12; we will identify each fricative reflex
set by its voiced member, *z* , *zh*, or *l*.

Table 12 The three basic fricatives and their reflexes.

Voiced reflex	Voiceless reflex	D-effect reflex
z [z]	s [s]	dz [ts]
zh [ʒ]	sh [ʃ]	j [tʃ]
l [l]	ł [ɬ]	dl [tl]

An examination the YM root/stem index shows that there is also a set of glide-initial stems. These glides have special properties. Take for instance the stem YóóD (g352). When this initial glide is in a voiceless environment, it surfaces as the coronal fricative and when it is in the context of a *d*-effect it surfaces as the affricate *dz*, as YM notes. Thus, this glide patterns like a *z* type [+ant] coronal fricative, except that it surfaces as a coronal glide in the voiced environment. An example of this alternation is in (23) and (24). The verb stem is listed as *YóóD* in the Root / Stem / Theme Index (g315), but it appears as *sóód* after the *sh* in (23), and *dzóód* after the *d*-of the 1st dual marking in (24).

(23)   hanis sóód

ha	# [n	ish	] [ø	yóód	]
'out'	# ['thematic'	øimp/1ˢᵗ	] ['cl'	'drive a small herd'	]
D	# [	Aux	] [	Verb	]

'I drive them (a small herd) out' (YM:d414)

(24)   hanii dzóód

ha	# [n	iid	] [ø	yóód	]
'out'	# ['thematic'	øimp/1ˢᵗdual	] ['cl'	'drive a small herd'	]
D	# [	Aux	] [	Verb	]

'We drive them (a small herd) out' (YM:d414)

Thus the pattern for this consonant is *y-s-dz*; the glide is its voiced reflex. We will refer to this segment as Yc, the coronal glide, in keeping with the convention of referring to a fricative in its voiced reflex. If we examine the entries in the Root / Stem / Theme Index we find that 3 out of the 53 Y-initial stems exhibit this alternation pattern: these stems begin with Yc fricatives.

There is a second alternation pattern for the Yc fricative, a *y-s-d* pattern, which shows up in one stem, the verb stem *yą́* 'eat'. According to YM87:g352, "In the presence of D-Classifier, stem-initial y- becomes d-, and *ł* classifier + y- = s-." The voiceless reflex can be seen in (25), and the d-effect reflex in (26).

(25)   bi'iis są́
       bi # ['   (y)i ish   ] [ł   yą́]
       'him' # [3iO ser. øimp/1ˢᵗ] ['cl' 'eat']
        D # [Aux   ] [Verb   ]
       'I made him eat' (YM:d215)

(26)   'áde'ash dą́
       'áde   # ['(a) ish   ] [d   yą́]
       'above self' # [3iO øimp/1ˢᵗ] ['cl' 'eat']
        D   # [Aux   ] [Verb   ]
       'I overeat (eat above oneself)' (YM:d12)

There is an additional dorsal fricative pattern that exhibits not only the three reflexes, but also 3 alternatives for the voiced reflex. This pattern occurs for the stem *YEED*, 'run' (g350); the form *yeed* is the imperfective, and *wo'* is the neuter form of the same stem. The stem-initial consonant is co-articulated with the following vowel, appearing as *y* before high front vowels, as in (27), and *w* before the round vowel, as in (28). In its voiceless reflex, the initial consonant appears as *h* [x], as seen in (29). The forms in (27), (28) and (29) are all listed under the stem entry for *YEED*.

(27)   dish yeed
       [d (y)ish] [l yeed]
       [Aux   ] [Verb]
       'I start to run along' (YM:g350)

(28)   dinish wo'
       [d nish] [l wo']
       [Aux   ] [Verb]
       'I am a fast runner' (YM:g350)

(29)   ha'nish heed
       ha # [' nish] [ł yeed]
        D # [Aux] [Verb]
       'I went lame' (YM:g350)

(30) shows yet another reflex that appears before the low vowel *a*: the initial segment of the verb stem *gháád* 'to shake, flap' (g328). I give two forms, with the voiced *gh* reflex in (30) and its voiceless *h* [x] reflex in (31).

(30)   yi gháád
       [yi   ] [gháád   ]
       [3ʳᵈ Su] ['move rapidly']
       [Aux] [Verb   ]
       'I'm shaking it' (YM:g328)

(31) yish háád
      [yish   ] [gháád   ]
      [1ˢᵗ Su] ['move rapidly']
      [Aux] [Verb   ]
      'He is shaking it' (YM:g328)

Finally, in (32), we see a form with the reflexive *'ádi*, which requires the *d*-classifier: the d-effect reflex is *g* for this velar consonant. Young and Morgan (1987:d24) gloss *'ádi* as a compound morpheme: (*'á # [d(i)*). It is glossed below as simply the reflexive.

(32) 'ádísh gáád
      'á di (i)sh   [d   gháád   ]
      reflex. 1ˢᵗ Su ['cl' 'move rapidly']
                      [Verb   ]
      'I'm shaking myself'

We will call this glide the back or Yd fricative. YM note that the symbol y is used to represent two different kinds of sounds, both a coronal glide *y*, and a 'voiced velar spirant' [ɣ]: the *w* represents the rounded version ɣ^w. The velar spirant is written as either *y, w* or *gh*, depending on the following vowel (These alternations are listed in a chart on page:xv.). In many speakers this segment has become lenited to an approximant more closely reflecting its orthographic representation, though it retains some constriction. We will examine the quality of this sound in Chapter 5.

Table 13 Fricatives (including glides) and their Reflexes.

Fricative Type	Stem-initial Consonant	'Voiced' Reflex	Voiceless Reflex	D-effect Reflex
Basic Fricatives	Z	z	s	dz [ts]
	ZH	zh [ʒ]	sh [ʃ]	j [tʃ]
	L	l	ł	dl [tł]
Glides	Yc	y	s	dz
	Yc	y	s	d
	Yd	y/w/gh	h	g

Thus there are two main sets of segments: stops which are stable in the phonology and do not undergo any alternations, and fricatives and approximants, which appear as one of three reflexes depending on the context. Table 13 provides a comprehensive chart of the six reflex sets we've discussed.

We will discuss the spectral properties of the coronal and dorsal glides in Chapter 5.

3.5   CONJUNCT ALTERNATIONS

Fricatives undergo a number of alternations in the conjunct domain, several of which are not apparently phonological. I will discuss some of more prominent of these alternations in this section.

3.5.1   The S-perfective

The s-perfective conjugation (g200-1) has an unusual property. The conjugation marker is *s*, but it only appears if the form is either word-initial or at the conjunct/disjunct boundary (g233ff). Otherwise, the form acts as if it were vowel initial. Note that (33) contains the word-initial sperfective/1st *sé*, while in (34) it is preceded by a conjunct prefix *d-^{1}*, the inceptive (d:331). The *d* appears in the onset of the form as *dé-*; we would expect **disé* if there were a fricative in the initial position of te s-perfective. In (35) the form *sé* is preceded by a disjunct prefix *'á*, but it is at the disjunct/conjunct boundary, so it is protected and surfaces as *sé*.

(33)   séł dzid
    [sé   ] [ł   dzid   ]
    [sperf/1st] ['cl' 'shake, agitate']
    [Aux   ] [Verb   ]
    'I shook it in a pan' (YM:d774)

(34)   dé dzíí'
    [d   sé   ] [d   dzíí'   ]
    [inceptive sperf/1st] ['cl' 'breath']
    [Aux   ] [Verb   ]
    'I took a breath' (YM:d331)

(35)   'áséł díịd
    'á # [sé   ] [ł   díịd   ]
    Ib # [sperf/1st] ['cl' 'disappear']
    D # [Aux] [Verb   ]
    'I got rid of it' (YM:g233,column 78)

In this way, the initial *s* segment of the s-perfective has some of the properties of the stem-initial consonant in the verb stem YÁ'; it surfaces as an *s* in the voiceless context (word-initial is a voiceless position (YM:g9)), or at the disjunct/conjunct boundary (c). However, when the s-perfective form is prefixed, the prefix appears in the onset.

3.5.2   The Qualifier Alternations

The Qualifer prefixes of Position VIc are the other consonantal alternation patterns we find among the prefix consonants. These are a difficult set of alternations. This position holds a series of y- prefixes, some of which alternate with *s*, some with the default vowel *i* and some with *h*. I refer the reader to YM (g:104) for discussion and examples. One thing to note is that many of the long vowels in the prefix domain (outside the Aux stem) are derived via the presence of one of these prefixes. I give examples below of the h-seriative, a Qu prefix of Pos VIa, as it appears as a prefix on the Aux stem in (36) and (37), with the ø-imperf/3rd and n-imperf/3rd respectively, and itself prefixed by an Agr *j* in (38) (the forms in (37) and (38) are constructed from the paradigm chart on page d445).

(36)   hi kę́ęs
    [h   i   ] [ø   kę́ęs   ]
    [ser. øimp/3rd] ['cl' 'move SSO']
    [Aux   ] [Verb   ]
    'to fall one after another(3rd Su)' (YM:d444)

(37)   hee chééh
    [h   í   ] [d   chééh]
    [ser. nimp/3rd] ['cl' 'hop']
    [Aux   ] [Verb   ]
    'to arrive hopping (3rd Su)' (YM:d445)

(38)   jiyee chééh
    [j   h (í)   ] [d   chééh]
    [3a ser. nimp/3rd] ['cl' 'hop']
    [Aux   ] [Verb   ]
    'someone arrives hopping'

The h-seriative appears as an *h* before the conjunct/disjunct boundary and as a glide *y* when it is prefixed by Agr. This is the general pattern of these Pos VIc prefixes: sensitivity to the disjunct /conjunct boundary, and alternation (either glide or vowel) when prefixed. I include them here because these alternation patterns mimic the ones found in the stems among the fricatives, and these can be given a phonological explanation. However, it is difficult if not impossible to separate out the paradigmatic variations (such as the *ee* in the forms (*h* + n-imp/3 → *hee*)) from what might be more purely phonological ones. I leave this to further work.

3.6   BOUNDARY EFFECTS

A 'boundary effect' is a phonological process that occurs only at the edge of a domain. In this instance, we refer conjunct/disjunct and stem/conjunct boundaries, as well as the right and left edge of a word. The effects fall into two major categories: segmental and prosodic. In this section we will discuss two of these effects: the alternations that occur on the stem-initial consonant (the classifier alternations and the 'd-effect') and the alternations that occur at the disjunct conjunct boundary.

3.6.1   The D-effect and Classifier Alternations

The best known and studied of the phonological patterns in Athabaskan is called the d-effect. It occurs at the important boundary between the stem and the conjunct domain. The d-effect is a set of alternations that occur on stem-initial segments across the Athabaskan language family. It has been discussed extensively in the literature (Sapir-Hoijer 1967, Stanley 1969, Howren 1971, Wright 1983, Bennet 1987, LaMontagne and Rice 1995, McDonough 2001). I will give an outline of the process here, referring the reader to the literature on the subject.

The alternation appears on stem-initial fricatives when they are adjacent to a *d*-segment, either the *d*-classifier or the d from *–iid,* a form of the 1st dual that consistently appears throughout the conjugations of the Base Paradigms. The mutations on the stem-initial fricatives are the source of the third set of fricative reflexes as discussed in Section 3.4. All the fricatives are affected (both the true fricatives and ones with glide reflexes in the voicing environment (recall Table 13)). In addition, the nasals and the glottal stop also exhibit *d*-effect alternations (n → 'n; ' → t').

While the segmental aspects of this alternation – the mutations on the stem-initial consonants – have received the majority of attention, the most interesting aspect of the pattern is in its prosody. The *d*-effect is part of a broader pattern which affects all the classifier prefixes: the lateral classifiers *l* and *ł* as well as the *d*-classifier. The stem as a morphological entity seems to disallow affixation that would put segmental material between itself and the domain boundary. This can be seen as a constraint, categorized simply as a constraint that aligns the morphological category 'stem' with the (morpho) boundary 'verb'. This alignment is governed by a couple of other principles: a recoverability constraint – keep the classifier - and a morpheme structure constraint –the output must accord with the segmental inventory. The maximum recoverability is accomplished by incorporating the classifier into the onset. This is what occurs with the *d*-classifier. Recall the *d* is an unaspirated coronal stop and the combination of *d* + fricative is an affricate, so the *d* segment adds a period of closure to the onset. This is Howren's insight, viewing the Athabaskan 'd-effect' as incorporation into the stem, as in (39).

(39) d + [CV]stem → [dCV]stem

Examples of this are in (40) through (43), showing the d segment with a central and lateral fricative, *z* and *l* respectively, in (41) and (43). These examples are taken from YM's section on the classifiers. In the d-effects, i.e. with the d-classifier, the stems surface with the affricates *dz* and *dl* respectively (41) and (43) (For discussion of the bi/yi alternation see XRF).

(40) yiih yiyíí ziid
      yiih   [yiyíí   ] [ø   ziid   ]
      'into it' [3rdO-yperf/3rd] ['cl' 'pour']
                [Aux   ] [Verb   ]
      'he poured it(into it)' (YM:g120)

(41) biih yi dziid
      biih   [yi   ] [d   ziid   ]
      'into it' [yperf/3rd] ['cl' 'pour']
                [Aux   ] [Verb   ]
      'he poured it(into it)' (YM:g120)

(42) yoo lóós
      [yoo   ] [ø   lóós   ]
      [3rdO-prog/3rd] ['cl' 'lead']
      [Aux   ] [Verb   ]
      'he is leading it along' (YM:g120)

(43) *yi dlóós*
      [yi   ] [d   lóós   ]
      [prog/3rd] ['cl' 'lead']
      [Aux   ] [Verb   ]
      'it is being lead along' (YM:g120)

The second part of this is the appearance of the classifiers in the coda of the second syllable. In (44) the lateral classifier appears as the coda of the penult syllable. If the penult syllable is closed, then the classifier may delete instead, as in (45).

(44) yíł ch'al
      [yí   ] [ł   ch'al   ]
      [sperf/3rd] ['cl' 'lap up']
      [Aux   ] [Verb   ]
      'I lapped it up' (YM:d779)

(45)   yish ch'al
       [(y)ish   ] [ɫ   ch'al   ]
       [øimp/3rd] ['cl' 'lap up']
       [Aux   ] [Verb   ]
       'I lap it up' (YM:d779)

Figure 6 diagrams some of the options for classifier expression. The incorporation of the classifiers into coda position in (a) and the deletion of the classifiers between two consonants (b) is straightforward, the latter analyzable as a commonplace repair strategy that deletes a medial consonant in a CCC cluster.

```
a.  CV   ] [C+CV..]        →  CVC]       [CV
b.  CVC ] [C+CV..]         →  CVC]       [CV
              ⇓
              ø

c.  CV(C) ][ C+V..]        →  CV(C)]     [CV
```

Figure 6 The Navajo 'Classifier Generalization'.

The lateral classifier is absorbed by z-initial stems, appearing with a voiceless reflex[4]. There are several constraints on this process: first this only occurs when the coda position is open, that is to say when the Aux stem is an open syllable. If the Aux stem has a coda as in (45) the classifier deletes. Second the *d*-classifier does not appear here, nor does the coda of the *-Ciid* Aux stem. This is framed as a coda constraint on Aux stems. The observation is that the classifier alternations including the d-effect alternations are a result of prosodic imperatives, so the segmental alternations are secondary effects.

3.6.2 Morphophonemic D/Aux Boundary Alternations

The disjunct / conjunct boundary is a juncture in the verb word that represents a break between the Aux domain and the disjunct domain. This juncture does not have the prominence of the conjunct or Aux / stem boundary, which is marked by a number of quite salient properties, as we've seen. The Aux / stem boundary is the primary juncture in the word, and its prominence is supported by the distinct phonetic characteristics of the two groups. The disjunct / conjunct boundary is a more subtle juncture, at least phonologically, marking an internal break in the prefix complex. It is nevertheless one of the two primary boundaries in the word, marking a division between two domains with distinct semantic and pragmatic properties (Sussman 2003), the disjunct and auxiliary. It also marks a boundary for a number of phonological and morphophonemic alternations.

These alternations have been discussed in Kari (1976:) using rewrite rules. An example is the 'ni absorption' rule in (46).

(46) CV + ni[→ Cv́

This rules reads that the *ni* conjunct prefix becomes a high tone when there is a prefix between it and the disjunct/conjunct boundary, as in (47). The rule does not apply (the *ni* surfaces) if the prefix is from the disjunct group. In fact the *ni* in question is the øimp/2nd, the only conjugation in which *ni* appears. In example (48) the ni surfaces at the # boundary when preceded by a disjunct prefix *na* 'around'.

(47)   shí chid
       [sh   ni   ] [ø   chid   ]
       [1st O øimp/2nd] ['cl' 'scratch']
       [Aux   ] [Verb   ]
       'you're scratching me' (YM:g113)

(48)   nanił té
       na   # [ni   ] [ł   té   ]
       'around' # [øimp/2nd] ['cl' 'carry (animate object)']
                     [Aux   ] [Verb   ]
       'you're carrying it around' (YM:g113)

In (47) *ni-* appears as high tone default vowel í when it is preceded by an Arg *sh-* '1stobj'. We will consider this a morphophonemic, and not a phonological alternation, a part of the ø-imperfective paradigm. Another alternation that is more likely phonological in nature is the *h*-seriative alternations, in which the *h*-seriative appears as an *h* at this juncture and a vowel elsewhere, as we saw in (36) – (38) above.

Many of the alternations at this boundary, like the *ni* absorption rule, are governed by some aspect of the morphosyntax. YM solves this problem by simply listing most prefix combinations as paradigms in the Model Paradigms of Appendix I (g215-256) (See Chapter 6.3.2 on how to use these paradigm charts). Thus, these alternations are considered paradigmatic. While a phonological analysis may be given for many of them, the fact that there are so few phonemic contrasts in this domain, in combination with the richness of the morphosyntactic specifications, means that there is a lack of a clearly defined distinction between phonologically and syntactically motivated processes. While a phonological analysis may be descriptively adequate, it may well be misleading for the generalizations it misses concerning the grammatical and paradigmatic nature of the alternations.

3.7   METATHESIS OF J-

The Pos. V 'deictic subject marker *j*- has a unique distribution pattern among the prefixes in the Aux domain. The *j*- morpheme has a special meaning, the so-called '4th person'; I refer the reader to the discussion of this morpheme in YM (g76-77). The *j*-metathesis is an interesting pattern because it is the single instance of a linear re-ordering among the conjunct morphemes, and because this reordering can be described phonologically. For this reason I will describe its phonological pattern, from YM (g77).

This morpheme is the most obviously consonantal of the Aux prefixes, in that it appears to resist epenthesis. Instead it either is incorporated as an onset as in the examples in (49) (with a more detailed gloss in (50)), or it appears as a coda, mimicking the distribution of the lateral classifiers. Like the other prefixes, it is also sensitive to the Aux/stem boundary. YM lists a full page of alternations that the *j*- morpheme undergoes (g77). The basic generalization is that it either appears in the onset of a vowel initial morpheme such as the Aux stem, or it appears as a coda, in which case it undergoes a metathesis. The various phonological reflexes of this morpheme are conditioned by the environment it appears in, onset or coda, and the consonant harmony constraints.

Its participation in harmony is optional when the Aux stem is involved, but it is not apparently optional in its interaction with other prefixes.

(49) dzizdiz   ~ jizdiz   she spun it (YM:g77)
         biih dziłmáás ~ biih jiłmáás   he's rolling it (as up a mountain)

In (50) it appears in its 'rightful' place as an Agr morpheme, a prefix on the Aux stem; it is optionally under the harmony constraint.

(50)   dzizdiz ~ jizdiz
          [j   iz   ] [ø   diz   ]
          [3a sperf/3rd] ['cl' 'spin']
          [Aux   ] [Verb   ]
          'she spun it' (YM:g77)

When there is another prefix in the complex (not the Aux stem) it metathesizes, as in (51). The *j*- appears in coda position, where it is under a coda constraint which bars affricates, and it surfaces as the fricative *zh*. This changes its position relative to the other prefix. In (51), the j- (Agr, pos V) appears after the h-seriative a Qualifier prefix of Pos VIa.

(51)   dihizhdi 'aah
        di   # [hi   j   d   i   ] [ø   'aah]
        'fire' # [ser. 3a theme øimp/3rd] ['cl' stem]
        Ib   # [VI   V   VI   VII/VIII] [IX   X   ]
         D   # [Aux   ] [Verb   ]
        'he's putting them one after another into or near the fire'

The nature of this metathesis has not been investigated, When it metathesizes, it takes the shapes *zh/z*. The metathesis apparently always is of this type: it metathesizes to the coda of a syllable of a prefix to the Aux stem. It does not metathesize with the Aux stem.

3.8   CONCLUSION

The phonological system in Navajo is characterized by two main patterns: the distinctive phonotactic constraints on phoneme distribution and the segmental alternations that fricatives undergo.   The phoneme distribution in Navajo is severely constrained.   Stems are phonotactically privileged, being the only place in the language where the full sets of contrasts occur; the phonemic inventory is basically a list of the stem onsets. Because of the morphological structure of the language, the constraint results in a striking limitation on the distribution of contrasts. We will see n the next chapter that distribution has an effect on segmental timing and duration profiles.   The conjunct or Aux and disjunct domains in the verb are areas of reduced contrasts, though one category of prefixes in the disjunct domain (Ib, the 'bound postpositionals') show some of the phonotactic properties of stems.   The inventory is coronal heavy, and consonant harmony further reduces the set of possible contrasts within a word.   Place of articulation in Navajo is not a robust contrast.   Syllable structure also distinguishes the stem from affixes, as stems have long vowels and codas, while prefixes are CV.   The CV syllable structure of the prefixes is an arguable result of the fact that these morphemes are underlyingly non-syllabic consonants attached to the stem.   The Aux stems are forms from the Base Paradigm conjugations (g200-1).

As for segmental phonology, the stops are inert.   The main alternations are undergone by the fricatives, which surface in stems as sets of three reflexes, determined by context, voiced, voiceless or 'd-effect'.   A second set of significant alternations are found among the classifiers.   These prefixes to the verb stem exhibit a set of alternations arguably due to prosodic phenomena; this analysis encompasses the *d*-effect alternations within it.   That is, the d-effect is part of a set of alternations undergone by the classifier prefixes to the verb stem.   In this view the verb stems appear to bar affixation, causing their prefixes, the classifiers, to surface in alternate ways determined by prosodic imperatives and governed by recoverability.

Finally, the fricatives undergo a number of sometimes elusive alternations in the conjunct domain, in particular in the s-perfective conjugation and with prefixes like as the *h*-seriative and the 4th person *j*-.

In the next chapters we will examine the results of a phonetic study of the sound system of Navajo.

---

[1] It is an interesting fact that the consonants of this conjunct domain are not much larger than the set of inflectional contrasts in English, {d, t, n, s, z} despite the considerable differences in the size and productivity of the inflectional morphology between these two languages.

[2] Given that other Athabaskan languages are argued to have noun incorporation, (Axelrod 1991) these incorporated postpositional stems are an interesting aspect of the disjunct domain and may represent an incorporation system that has lost its productivity. See the discussion of postpositional stems in YM (g26-35)

[3] The default vowel differs across the language family. In other Athabaskan languages such as Salcha (Tuttle and Hargus 1996) it is the neutral vowel schwa, for instance. One question that comes to mind is the relationship, if any, between the default vowel specification and metrical stress. Do the Athabaskan languages that have metrical stress tend to have a reduced default vowel?

[4] YM note this in their dictionary entries as (ł + ziid → siid).

Chapter 4

DURATION AND TIMING

4.0   INTRODUCTION

In describing of the profile of the speech patterns of a community, segmental duration is a revealing aspect of the sound system (Lehiste 1970, Klatt 1976). Quantitative duration differences serve a function at every level in the grammar, from syllable (vowels are longer before voiced consonants in English) to utterance level (final lengthening). The implementation of local differences in duration mark a wide range of phenomena: in the realization of metric structure and stress, of prosodic position-in-word and -utterance, focus and intonation, markedness, and extra-linguistic phenomena such as speech rate. Duration is a quantitative measure explicitly associated with different phonological, prosodic and psychological phenomena, making it one of the more problematic aspects of an interface between phonetics and phonology. In the same vein, duration effects are also to a large degree language specific. In many languages with metric stress systems, unstressed vowels are shorter than stressed ones, but the implementation of that reduction vary cross-linguistically (Lehiste 1970, Crosswhite 2001). That is to say, duration, while quantitative, is not determined by purely physiological phenomena. This means that specific information about duration and lengthening must be encoded in the implementation of lexical representations. In particular, because of the close association of lengthening with the expression of metric stress, pitch accent and prosodic features like intonation and focus, the prosodic organization of a language will be explicitly reflected to one extent or another in its duration profile, in a similar way that a pitch contour reflects tonal structure.

In this chapter I will investigate duration and timing effects in Navajo. The task is to provide a baseline profile of the Navajo word, by examining the timing patterns of the verbal domains within the word and the details of those domains, as an expression of its organization.

As we saw in Chapter 3, there is a strong phonotactic bias in the distribution of segment types in the word. The phonemic inventory is, in large part, a list of the stem onsets and nuclei. Outside this position the contrasts are quite reduced: the set of contrasts in the conjunct and disjunct domains is a small set of mostly simple coronal consonants and default vowels. This means that the full set of phonemic contrasts is confined to a single position in the word: in the stem, which is at the right edge of the verb. In all verbs, which are minimally bisyllabic, and most nouns, which have prefixes, the right most morpheme is not in a word-initial position. Thus, most of the phonemic contrasts in Navajo, which are confined to stem onsets, only appear inside a word, seldom occurring at an edge. As such, most segmental contrasts are in comparatively stable positions. Since the Athabaskan languages are prefixal, and the prefixes have reduced inventories, only a reduced number of phonemes occur in word-initial position, where a segment is more likely to exhibit an observable variability in articulation. This distribution fact implicates a relationship between what several linguists have referred to as the 'rigidity' of the Athabaskan word, its prosodic structure and its phonetic implementation.

The term rigidity as applied to Athabaskan is generally used to mean that the order of morphemes is fixed in the word and, classically, that morpheme concatenation must model this fixed ordering. But the rigidity in the verb has implications that extend beyond morpheme ordering. It means, for one, that there are likely to be powerful distributional constraints at play at every level of the grammar; the richer the morphology, that is the more information that is encoded in the morphology, the more far-reaching the distributional constraints are likely to be. We have seen these constraints at work in the phonotactics of the verb. Since the verb is a major part of the vocabulary, the patterns internal to the verb are likely to be some of the major sound patterns in the language. They undoubtedly play a major role in the shape of the lexicon, and the profile of the verb word is likely to have an influence in defining a community's overall speech patterns. A description of the verb-internal patterns is the groundwork for understanding of the speech patterns in the language. This chapter is a study of the relationship of the phonotactics to segmental timing and duration.

In this chapter we will examine the details of timing and duration and their function within the verb, beginning with an examination of the properties that are associated with each of the three domains in the verb. Then we will examine the duration properties that occur within each domain.

4.1   DOMAIN DURATIONS

This section will investigate the duration of the individual domains in the verb, focusing on how each contributes to the total duration of the verb word. Recall that the three domains have different phonotactic properties and are marked by boundaries in distinct ways. The verb stem is a single syllable (and is congruent with the Verb domain, I use the terms Stem and Verb interchangeably here[1]), the conjunct domain is at least one syllable and may contain two or three syllables, and although the disjunct domain is optional, it may contain two or more morphemes. The disjunct and conjunct domains are alike in that, apart from the morphemes of the disjunct position Ib, whose morphemes YM call postpositional stems, they are domains of largely reduced contrasts and default specifications.

Table 14 shows the base statistics for the duration measurements for the verb and its domains. These measurements were calculated across a 32 word dataset (1st column, row 1), containing 112 syllables (2nd column, row 1) and 14 speakers. The table reports the median, standard deviation, range and interquartile range (IQR = mid 50%) of the words in the data set, each of the three domains in the word, and the Conjunct and Stem domain combined. The 32 words in the data base include 21 Disjunct domains (21 of the 32 words in the data set had Disjunct domains), and 32 of the Conjunct and the Stem domains (since every verb has both a conjunct and a stem domain).

Table 14 Median word and domain duration measurements in ms.

	Count	(Syllable counts)	Median	St.Dev.	Range	IQR
Word	32	(112)	1167.8	242.3	1074.4	310.1
Disjunct	21	(28)	232.1	120.9	611.1	111.9
Conjunct	32	(54)	508.1	156.8	567.0	266.4
Stem	32	(32)	502.3	153.1	537.3	256.8
Conj+Stem	32	(86)	967.9	191.7	818.4	254.4

The three domains contribute to the duration of the word in distinct ways. First, observe the contribution that the conjunct and stem domains make to the average duration of the word across the dataset. The median, standard deviation, and interquartile range (IQR) for the stem and conjunct domains is about the same, although the number of syllables that the durations were calculated across were different (conj = 54, stem = 32). On average the conjunct and stem domains contribute equally to the duration of the word in this dataset. Contrast this with the statistics for the Disjunct domain. We can see this illustrated in the boxplot in Figure 7. The durations of the Conjunct, Stem and Conjunct + Stem domains are plotted in the last three columns.

For each of the five categories Word, Disjunct, Conjunct, Stem, and Conjunct + Stem, Figure 7 shows the median of the data values in this dataset (the line across the box), the spread of the data by IQR for each category (the box), and symmetry of the distribution of the data values around the median (the shaded area). Finally, extreme outliers are marked (one in the disjunct domain). The edges of the box are the mid 50% of the

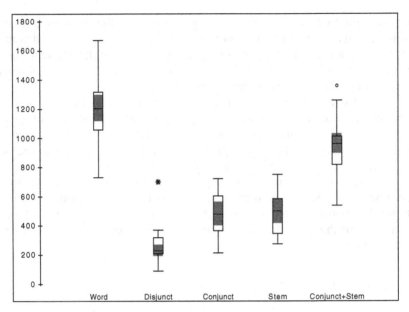

Figure 7 Boxplots of the word and domain durations of the Navajo verbs in the dataset.

data (the IQR), and the whiskers mark the full range of the data, barring the extreme values.

Observe that even though the ratio of the stem-to-conjunct durations across the data are approximately even, the stem syllables only make up about 41% of the syllables in the conjunct + stem data combined. In the data, an averaged stem syllable is about 40% (184 ms) longer than an averaged conjunct syllable. Note that this is a statement about the domain averages, and not individual syllables within the dataset; word length will vary according the number and kind of syllables in the word, and the segmental make-up of those syllables. This conjunct/stem ratio indicates that these domains on average equally contribute to the duration of the word in this dataset, independent of the number of syllables counted in the average. The box plots demonstrate this. That is to say, the three domains reflect different duration patterns. Another way to see this is to examine the syllable count patterns.

The difference in the duration patterns in the three domains in the verb can be seen as a ratio score. Table 15 provides a syllable score for each domain calculated by taking the overall domain duration average (mean in ms: 276.3 disjunct, 475.5 conjunct, 491.5 stem) and dividing it by the number of syllables counted in that average. This gives us a figure that reflects the contribution a domain specific syllable is likely to make to the duration of the word as a whole. The results are scores of 9.5 for the disjunct, 8.8 for the conjunct and 15.6 for the stem. In this way the syllable score is a measure of the differences in the duration patterns among the domains[2].

Table 15 Syllable score for each domain in the verb. The syllable score is the mean domain duration divided by the number of syllables.

	Disjunct	Conjunct	Verb Stem
Syllable score	9.5	8.8	15.6

All things being equal, we might expect the number of syllables in a domain to have a direct influence on its syllable score. The word would vary in duration directly dependent on the number of syllables in the word: more syllables, incrementally longer duration. Thus in this data the conjunct domain, with the greatest number of syllables, would be the longest domain on average, followed by the disjunct, then the stem which is always only a single syllable, as the shortest. This is not the case (see Table 14): the duration differences between these domains do not correspond to the differences in the syllable counts in the domains. The conjunct domain ought to be larger than the stem domain by a much greater degree than it is; the disjunct also ought to be longer than the stem. The stem domain has the highest syllable score, followed by the disjunct. The conjunct domain syllables are compressed in comparison to both the stem and to a lesser degree the disjunct. What factors account for this phenomena?

There are several factors that come into play. One obvious concern is the position of the Verb stem. It is at the right edge of the word and, since the words were spoken in isolation, stems are also utterance final. As such, they are perhaps subject to utterance final lengthening effects, of the type found in other languages, most notably in English (Beckman and Edwards 1990). Prosodically driven lengthening above the level word in the grammar, such as final lengthening, may well play a role in the language, as we will discuss. We will consider this in the next section when we take a closer look at the duration properties of segments within the domains. However, final lengthening is unlikely to be a complete explanation for the stem's high syllable score, since the disjunct domain also has a larger score than the conjunct domain. One explicit difference between the disjunct and conjunct domains is the presence of stem-like morphemes in the disjunct domain, the postpositional stems. These morphemes have phonotactic properties congruent to stems. If this phonotactic semblance can be reasonably argued to account for the difference in the scores of the disjunct versus conjunct domain, then the phonotactic properties have a determining effect on domain length and by extension on the verb's duration patterns.

Is the conjunct domain score smaller simply because of kinds of syllables found in this domain differ from those found in the stems? That is to say, is there a syllable type effect?

This does not overtly seem to be the case. Stems have both long vowels and codas. But this is true for both the Verb stem and the Aux stem in the conjunct domain. Both the conjunct and verb stem domains in this data tended to have the same number of domain-final codas (24 conjunct / 27 stems), although the stems tended to have more long vowels (23/32 for stems, 10/54 for conjunct). This distribution fact is not an artifact of the data, however, but reflects a clear phonotactic pattern in the language. Only the stems have the full set of contrasts, both consonantal and vocalic. In the conjunct domain when there are long vowels, they tend to be either paradigmatic (i.e. in the "Base" or Mode paradigms of YM:200) or derived over a boundary (disjunct/conjunct). Thus stems have more contrasts than the conjunct morphemes and tend to have more long vowels. This may be a contributing factor in the syllable score differences between the conjunct and stem domains, but it does not account for the pattern since the conjunct score was also lower than the disjunct score which had fewer numbers of syllables and both fewer long vowels and no codas in those syllables.

Another consideration is the fact that the closure period on word-initial stops was not measured. Since stems are never word-initial, this may mitigate against the even conjunct/stem ratio in the duration facts.Again, this is unlikely to be the cause of the distinction in syllable scores, since not all words began with conjunct boundary, and those that did were not consistently stop-initial.

Where do these ratios come from?Are they a legitimate reflection of the organization of the word, or are they epiphenomenal? In answering these questions in the next sections, we will examine the durations of the consonants and vowels within the domains of the word independently. Also, since duration is the one of the primary means by which metric stress is realized, we ought to be able to detect the presence of metric phenomena in systematic patterns of duration measurements among the alternating syllables of the word.

4.2   DURATION PATTERNS IN THE STEMS

This section and the next will investigate the duration profile of consonants in the three domains, beginning in this section with the duration factors of stem consonants in nouns and verbs, while section 4.3 will look at the duration of consonants in the disjunct and conjunct domains. Finally, in section 4.4, we'll turn our attention to vowel durations.

4.2.1 Stem Consonant Durations

The two principle types of grammatical categories in the morphology are prefixes and stems. In this section we will consider the properties of stems.There are three types of stems in the grammar: noun stems, verb stems and the Aux stems, the forms that comprise the Base Paradigms of

Young and Morgan (g200-1). I'll discuss these stem types separately in later subsections, but will begin here with some general features common to all of these stem types.

A confluence of factors conspires to make stems prominent morphemes in the word. They are marked by properties that distinguish them from prefixes, both in their specific phonotactic and syllable structure and their rigid distribution on the right edge of their domain, as the head of that domain. One question that arises is the nature of that prominence. We expect structurally defined features, like stress, to have consistent acoustic correlates. Do the verbs exhibit any diagnostics of structurally assigned prominence? Can, for instance, the bisyllabicity of the verb be analyzed as a foot- or prosodically based phenomena? While there is no direct correspondence between any acoustic feature and stress or meter, it is well known that duration has a major role in expressing these structural phenomena. To this purpose we will examine the timing relationships in the segments and syllables.

The category 'stem' in Navajo is a monosyllable of the shape CV(V)(C). The minimal syllable size in Navajo is the open syllable (CV), but stems vowels may be long and the syllables may be closed. Though nouns are less common than verbs in the Navajo lexicon, nouns have a much simpler structure than verbs. We used (mainly) nouns to examine the consonantal and vocalic contrasts of the segment inventory, and the verbs to investigate the domain level groups. The verb word list was set up to show a variety of types of complex words; the concern was less with purely segmental issues. We will discuss the nouns and verbs separately, starting with the stem-initial contrasts in nouns. For the greater part, in the noun stems, the consonants were measured intervocalically, in a VCV context.

Figure 8 is a spectrogram of the Navajo word *bita'* [pɪtxɑʔ], 'his father' (bi+ta'), from a female speaker. There are several aspects of this spectrogram worthy of note. The timing profile of the noun-stem onset that we see here is characteristic of the stem-initial stop consonants in general. We will take this topic up in a separate section on stop consonants (Section 4.2.3). Also observe the steady state of the vowel formants, as well as the sharp onset and offset of the consonant articulation and vowel formants. These are characteristic of the Navajo speech signal and they make segmentation of Navajo speech straightforward. Note also the difference in the duration of the two syllables of this noun token. Both vowels in the noun are short vowels, but the first is a prefix vowel; prefix vowels are often extremely reduced in the nouns, a characteristic of prefix-noun words. Note that the final vowel is closed with a weakening of the vowel gestures into aspiration. We see in the data that the final vowel of open syllables in Navajo are closed with either this type of aspiration or by a glottal stop or glottalization. These gestures tend to occur somewhat independently of the actual orthographic representation of the syllable as a open or closed with a glottal stop; that is to say glottalization varies between a full stop and creaky

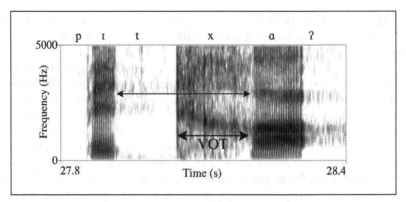

Figure 8 Spectrogram of the Navajo word *bita'* [pɪtxɑʔ]. The duration of the
aspirated coronal stop *t* is indicated by the top arrow.

voice and this is true of both CV and CVʔ syllables. The words with an
orthographic final *h* more consistently appear with aspiration. Finally,
relevant to the present discussion, note the length of the intervocalic
consonant *t* [tx]; this is an aspirated coronal stop, marked by the top arrow in
the spectrogram. YM classify this segment as an affricate (YM:xiii),
however the length of this stem-initial stop, its closure-to-release ratio and
the heaviness and duration in the release period are characteristics of Navajo
stop consonants in general (McDonough and Ladefoged 1994). We will
take up a discussion of stops below in Section 4.2.3.

Finally, in a discussion of the structure of phonemic inventories
Linblom and Maddieson (1988) make a distinction between simple,
elaborated and complex segments which is relevant to the present
investigation. Their paper is an attempt to define the concept of a perceptual
space for consonants and consonant inventories; the idea is that the
development of complex inventories is not random. Inventories develop
elaborated and complex segments only after a basic inventory space of
simple segments has been saturated. The need to maintain perceptual
distinctions regulates an inventory's complexity. Their definition of
complexity is articulatory; a simple segment is a simple gesture, an
elaborated one is a combination of simple gestures, and complex segments
are more complex articulations. They give aspiration on a lateral affricate as
an example of a complex segment. In this view, Navajo has a complex
inventory. The Athabaskan inventory is clearly divided along two lines, as
we will see: the simple gestures of fricatives, nasals, unaspirated stops and
most glides, and the elaborated and complex segments which are
constructed by combining the simple gestures in constrained ways. The
stem onset in Figure 8, the aspirated coronal stop *t* [tx], is clearly a
combination of two 'simple' gestures: a stop closure, followed by a fricative
release which is strongly co-articulated with the following vowel. This
closure-release footprint is characteristic of all the stops in Navajo, except
for the unaspirated ones, which pattern with the fricatives in having more

basic footprints, i.e. they are comprised of simpler gestures. This point is of interest because it links the rigidity of morpheme order in Athabaskan to its phonotactics and to the size and type of its inventory. As we have noted, the rigidity results in the severe constraints on the distribution of contrasts in Athabaskan, where minimal pairs are rare, with most contrasts only occurring in stem onsets. Given these distributional constraints, one fundamental way to build functional contrast is to increase the complexity of the onset.

It is possible, of course, to talk of the complex segments as a combination of two distinct segments, that is, a consonant cluster (ts = t + s), but this characterization is superfluous since this onset is the only place these gestures combine in this way; there is no way to distinguish between a complex onset sound like an affricate and a cluster of two segments, except by definition. In addition these combinations themselves exhibit laryngeal contrasts (ts^h, ts'). The structure of stem onsets are not so much defined by syllable structure constraints, as they are by a constraint on the allowable complexity of a stem onset[3]. I will argue that the duration facts provide evidence that the onsets are best understood as a series of timing and sequencing constraints on licensed gestures, separate from the syllable structure constraints.

4.2.2 Duration Measurements in Nouns

The nouns consist of a stem, which is usually monosyllabic, and a prefix such as *bi* 'his/hers', the 3rd person singular prefix. About 80% of the nouns are of this form[4]. The remainder have other prefixes, or disyllabic stems, or, in a few cases, are verbal forms. All the consonants in prefix-noun sets are intervocalic. In the phonemic inventory there are two main types of consonants: the stop series, including the central and lateral affricates, and the continuants, the fricatives, nasals and glides. The fricatives are the most straightforward; they involve a constriction in the vocal tract that is held over the duration of the segment.

The fricatives as a series exhibit contextual variation that has been most commonly described as voiced and voiceless. The duration of the fricatives and nasals in the noun stems are listed in Table 16. I have included in this group the glottalized nasal '*m* [ʔm], as a reflex of the bilabial nasal, though it could also be considered in the stop group.

Voiceless fricatives *s* [s], *sh* [ʃ], and *ł* [ɬ] tend to be longer than their voiced reflexes, *z* [z] , *zh* [ʒ], and *l* [l], though there are no statistically significant duration differences between any of the fricatives. The nasal is the shortest segment (108 ms (37.3 St. dev)), however the coronal nasals *n* and '*n* were atypical in that they were not in intervocalic position in the dataset, but rather preceded by a coda *sh*. On average, the durations of consonants that are preceded by codas tend to be shorter than intervocalic consonants (section 4.1), so the status of the nasal as the shortest segment may have more to do with context in the data set than any intrinsic properties. The table shows the segments written in Navajo orthography in the first column (in italics) and their representation using the symbols of the IPA (the International Phonetic Alphabet) in the second column. The median, standard deviation, the range of the data, the IQR (the mid 50% of the data range) and count are also reported.

Table 16   Duration measurements of stem-initial fricatives and nasals in intervocalic position in nouns.

YM Orth.	IPA	Median	St.Dev.	Range	IQR	Count
s	s	208.8	74.0	319.6	75.6	29
z	z	177.5	42.3	146.4	67.2	23
sh	ʃ	208.6	39.1	148.8	56.5	16
zh	ʒ	179.1	34.4	102.6	45.3	7
ł	ɬ	158.4	55.3	212.2	92.1	20
l	l	140.9	50.3	180.7	70.6	17
h	x	129.6	62.3	281.7	89.2	39
n	n	108.0	37.3	105.9	65.4	16
m	m	138.5	25.5	79.1	28.0	7
'm	ʔm	233.0	103.0	336.4	112.7	8

I did not report the figures for the glottalized coronal nasal 'n because it was produced as a regular (non-glottalized) nasal by several of the speakers; there were only three 'n [ʔn] tokens in the dataset, lasting between 125 and 160 ms. Whether the production of this sound as a simple nasal n was due to the fact that it was not in intervocalic position, or because speakers do not produce glottalized coronal nasals, is unknown. Speakers did produce very clear examples of glottalized labial nasals 'm [ʔm], which was the longest segment (233 ms) reported in the chart in Table 16, and similar to the segments of the stops series in duration. The glottalized nasal is not properly an ejective with simultaneous oral and glottal closure, but, as Sapir (1929) first noted, a nasal consonant preceded by glottal gesture. Figure 9 is an example spectrogram of the glottalized nasal in the word yii'mas [ji:ʔmɑs].

The spectrograms are taken from the speech of two female speakers. The [ʔm] sequence in each is indicated by an arrow. These glottalized nasals exhibit the tendency of more complex segments to be longer than simple ones (section 4.2). The difference in duration between the speakers is primarily due to speech rate, which could not be controlled for because of the way the recording session was set up[5]. The speaker with the 317 ms onset had a tendency to speak quite slowly and clearly. In both

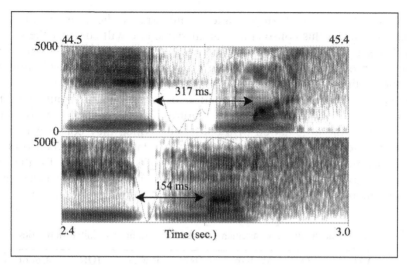

Figure 9 Spectrograms of the glottalized nasal *'m* (arrows) in the word *yii'mas*: two female speakers.

spectrograms, the articulation of the nasal consonant is clearly preceded by a glottal gesture, though the duration of the closure of the glottal gesture is quite different the two speakers. In both speakers, too, the glottal closure is preceded and followed by the glottal striations of creaky voice, though, again, the extent of this glottalization varies by speaker.

In Table 17 are the duration measurements for the stops series; these are segments which involve closure in the vocal tract. These include the plain stops (*b* [p], *d* [t], *t* [tx], *t'* [t'], *g* [k], *k* [kx], *k'* [k']) and the central (*dz* [ts], *ts* [tsʰ], *ts'* [ts'], *j* [tʃ], *ch* [tʃʰ], *ch'* [tʃ']) and lateral (*dl* [tɬ], *tl* [tɬʰ], *tl'* [tɬ']) affricates. The fricatives tend to be shorter on average than the stops as a class (179 / 232.2 ms). However, the affricates are significantly longer than the plain stops (170.8 / 236.8 ms). The unaspirated stops are on average the shortest segments in the table, while the ejective and aspirated affricates are the longest. The plain unaspirated stops and the fricatives are similar in duration (median: 170 / 179 ms).

Note that the glottalized nasal *'m* [ʔm] at 233 ms is the same length as the affricated stops. Thus we see a duration increase in the onset according to the complexity of the onset: simple continuants and unaspirated stops are the shortest, whereas the affricates and aspirated consonants tend to be longer.

Figure 10 demonstrates some of the differences between these groups. The three spectrograms are examples of an intervocalic nasal, stop, and fricative, *n t, s,* in stem-initial position in the words *binii', biteeł', bizid.* Each window is approximately 455 ms long. The nasal is 160 ms, the aspirated *t* is 303 ms, and the fricative is 180 ms. Note the longer duration of the aspirated coronal stop *t* [tx] as compared to the nasal and fricative, and the release portion of the consonant. This is a characteristic pattern for the aspirated coronal stop *t* and demonstrates the reason for YM's classification of this consonant as an affricate (we will consider the spectral qualities of this aspiration in Chapter 5). I have chosen to represent aspiration on the plain stops as a fricative [tx], rather than aspiration as a feature of the stop [t^h]. In a discussion of aspiration in stops, Ladefoged and Maddieson (1996) makes a distinction between two different ways that aspiration is used as a contrastive feature, as an aspect of the vocal fold vibration in the articulation of a consonant, which they consider to be its primary use, or, alternatively, as a timing relationship between oral and laryngeal gestures. Navajo uses both types of aspiration, but for the plain stops in Navajo, aspiration is clearly of the second sort (as we can see in the spectrogram in Figure 10), best characterized as a timing relationship.

Table 17 The duration measurements for the intervocalic stem-initial stop series.

YM	IPA	Median	St.Dev.	Range	IQR	Count
b	p	156.2	16.7	45.8	27.8	7
d	t	166.9	23.9	67.0	34.0	7
t	tx	230.5	31.2	90.2	32.3	7
t'	t'	252.7	27.6	97.3	41.8	11
g	k	133.5	25.1	72.2	35.1	7
k	kx	238.2	49.8	152.3	52.8	7
k'	k'	182.4	31.0	72.5	59.1	6
kw	kw	134.4	38.0	106.6	56.1	7
dz	ts	188.7	17.2	50.6	24.2	7
ts	ts^h	210.3	29.8	84.1	14.7	6
ts'	ts'	281.3	28.3	59.2	48.5	5
j	tʃ	178.1	18.4	48.8	27.1	7
ch	tʃ^h	235.4	14.7	41.7	21.7	7
ch'	tʃ'	228.6	31.4	87.4	48.6	7
dl	tɬ	230.8	40.8	107.0	58.3	7
tl	tɬ^h	255.9	31.5	86.4	49.9	7
tl'	tɬ'	280.1	55.6	132.2	106.0	8

Aspiration on the affricates *ts* [ts^h], *ch* [tʃ^h], *tl* [tɬ^h], is a different matter, perhaps necessarily, and may be best understood as aspiration in its more common interpretation, as a feature of vocal fold vibration (see Chapter 5.3.4). The aspiration of affricates as a aspect of vocal fold vibration will be examined in the next chapter.

All the stops, excepting the unaspirated ones but including the glottalized nasal, are complex segments, a combination of a series of gestures which constitute a characteristic footprint indicating a particular

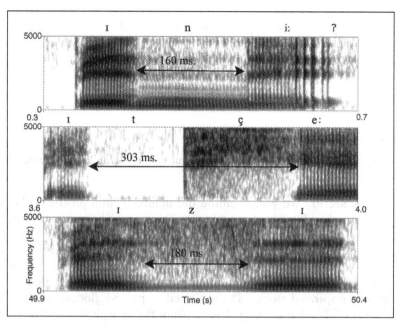

Figure 10 Spectrograms demonstrating the nasal *n*, stop *t* ([tx]), and fricative *z*, in stem initial position in the words *binii', biteeł, bizid*.

timing profile of oral and laryngeal articulations. We will take up a discussion of the duration profile of the stop series in the next section.

4.2.3 The Stem Stops

In the phonemic inventory, there are three kinds of stops: plain, affricated and laterally released. All the stops but the bilabial stop b [p], exhibit a three way laryngeal contrast as noted, exhibiting unaspirated, aspirated and ejective or glottalized variants. As we saw demonstrated in the spectrograms in Figure 10, most of the stop consonants have two distinct parts, a closure period followed by a release period before the start of the voicing of the vowel and the onset of the vowel formants.

In examining the stop contrasts in stem-initial position, I have taken independent duration measurements of both the stop closure and release period of the consonant, as Figure 11 demonstrates. The period from the release of the burst to the onset of voicing is called the voice onset time (VOT) for the purpose of this study, so that we may address the closure-release ratio and the nature of the releases in stops. The duration of the stop is the sum of these two measurements. Inherent to this definition is the notion that, for these consonants, VOT is a timing feature important in differentiating the stop gestures (Lisker and Abramson 1964, 1971, Browman and Goldstein 1990).

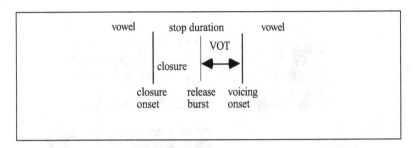

Figure 11 The divisions used in measurements of closure and release period (=VOT) in stops and affricates.

In this section we will examine the nature of this profile. The VOT durations for the plain stops are given in Table 18. The unaspirated bilabial and coronal stops have VOT's that are basically the size of the release burst (see Figure 17), though the VOT of the velar unaspirated stop is a little longer. As McDonough and Ladefoged (1992) pointed out, despite the orthographic representation of these stops as *b, d, g*, it is clear that they are voiceless unaspirated stops. The aspirated stops and glottalized stops have quite long VOT's that are very distinct from the unaspirated stops. There is a small difference between the VOT's of the aspirated and the ejective stops, the ejective VOT's being slightly shorter.

Table 18 Mean VOT of Navajo plain and affricated stops in ms with standard deviations in parentheses (from McDonough and Ladefoged 1992).

Plain		Unaspirated	Aspirated	Glottalized
	bilabial	12 (5)		
	coronal	6 (2)	130 (29)	108 (31)
	velar	45 (9)	154 (43)	94 (21)
Affricated				
	alveolar	91 (20)	149 (12)	142 (41)
	alveolo-palatal	68 (19)	153 (17)	144 (24)
	lateral	42 (20)	149 (29)	157 (40)

The major point to note is the magnitude of the VOT in the aspirated and glottalized stops as compared to the unaspirated plain stops. Navajo follows the phonetic tendency in many languages for velar stops to have a longer VOT than stops made at more anterior positions. The unaspirated velars are longer than the unaspirated coronals by about 40 ms. The difference in VOT between the aspirated velars and coronals is in the same direction, though smaller. The VOT of unaspirated bilabials are only 6 ms longer than the unaspirated coronals.

VOT measurements for the affricated stops are shown in the bottom half of Table 18. Again, the main point to observe in this table is that many of these releases are very long. The VOT for the velar ejective is more than double that reported by Lindau (1984) for the comparable stop in Hausa, and the coronal ejective is even longer. There are also a number of particular points of interest. In the alveolar and alveolo-palatal affricates by far the majority of the fricative release is voiceless. As we noted above, these measurements are from the stop release to the onset of voicing, so these measurements include the central or lateral fricative. An alternative definition of VOT might have entailed measuring from the release of the fricative to the onset of voicing, but we found it difficult to make reliable determinations of the moment when the fricative articulation could be said to be released. The fricative energy usually faded away as the vowel began. As in the plain stops, the aspirated and glottalized affricated stops are distinct from the unaspirated affricated stops. But in the case of these stops there is no difference between the VOT's of the aspirated and the ejective stops.

I suggest that in considering the consonantal contrasts in Navajo, a division between simple segments and complex segments is instructive in describing and understanding the timing characteristics of those contrasts in onsets. Onsets that are comprised of simple segments are shorter than those with complex segments; in Navajo complex segments are best understood in terms of a timing relationship between two (or more) kinds of gestures that are licensed by the phonotactics. Complex segments are composite gestures with a distinct timing relationship. The affricates and the aspirated and ejective stops are complex segments. The alternative is to treat the laryngeal contrasts as an aspect of the vocal fold vibration in the articulation of a plain or affricated stop. However, this characterization misses the generalization illustrated by the distinct and striking timing profiles of the complex segments, as well as the distinction between this timing relationship and contrasts that can be classified as more purely laryngeal, such as aspiration on affricates. This point bears discussion.

If a complex stem onset in Navajo has a closure period, it is coronal or velar. The bilabial consonants are confined to a small handful of morphemes and involve a simple closure gesture; its release is immediately followed by the articulation of the vowel. Thus the main portion of the distinctions between all but the unaspirated stops are found in the release periods. Therefore, consonantal distinctions fall into two main groups: the unaspirated plain stops b [p], d [t] and g [k], which have very short VOT's (basically the size of their release burst), and the aspirated and ejective plain stops and the central and lateral affricate series, all which have VOT's that are around 50% of the length of the consonant, as we can see in Figure 12. Table 19 shows the closure durations of both the plain and the affricated stops.

The unaspirated stops have longer closures (mean 132 ms, S.D. 36.5) than the aspirated stops (mean 96 ms, S.D. 23.0). Aspiration in these stops is quite fricated, as we can see in the spectrogram in Figure 8. The heaviness of the frication is a characteristic of the articulation of all aspirated and fricated consonants in the stem onset. The glottalized stops are not significantly different in closure duration from either of the other two types of stops. In addition, we should note that many of these closure durations are very long. Young and Morgan (1986:xv) have remarked that the consonants of Navajo are doubled between vowels; but it is the case that consonant gemination is not contrastive, i.e., the stops act like single complex segments.

Table 19 Mean closure duration of unaffricated and affricated stops in ms with standard deviations in parentheses.

Plain		Unaspirated		Aspirated		Glottalized	
	bilabial	154	(18)				
	coronal	162	(22)	118	(11)	149	(41)
	velar	102	(22)	97	(15)	76	(29)
Affricated							
	alveolar	98	(15)	62	(5)	121	(14)
	alveolo-palatal	101	(21)	84	(16)	98	(17)
	lateral	147	(42)	112	(15)	119	(33)

Figure 12 illustrates another way of considering the stop consonants in Navajo by showing the ratio between the stop's closure period and the duration of the stop as a whole. For most of the stops, except the unaspirated stops *b, d, g* [p, t, k], the VOT makes up near half of the duration of the consonant. Note also the difference in the bar graph between the plain coronals *d, t, t'* [t, tx, t'], and the affricated coronals *dz, ts, ts'* [ts, tsʰ, ts']. There is a sharp difference in VOT between the unaspirated coronal stop [t] and the aspirated and ejective coronal stops [tx, t']. But in the affricated series, the difference between [ts] and [tsʰ, ts'] is smaller. This difference between the two series is influenced by the fact that the affricate measurement includes the fricated release by definition. McDonough and Ladefoged (1992) note that they could not reliably measure the aspiration on the affricated stops, and the same is true of the more recent data. That is to say it was difficult to measure a voiceless interval which did not involve oral or pharyngeal frication between the release of the consonant and the onset of the vowel in the affricates. We will return to this in the next chapter.

The laterally released stops are somewhat different. In the unaspirated lateral plosive the voicing starts during the lateral. McDonough & Ladefoged (1992) point out that these sounds may not be affricates, but a combination of a stop + lateral fricative. Since the phonology does not make a distinction between affricates and stop + fricative sequences, nothing rests on this. However, given the pervasiveness of the d-effects throughout Athabaskan (where a d-segment is incorporated into a fricative initial onset, resulting in a stop + fricative sequence) the issue of the structure of the stem

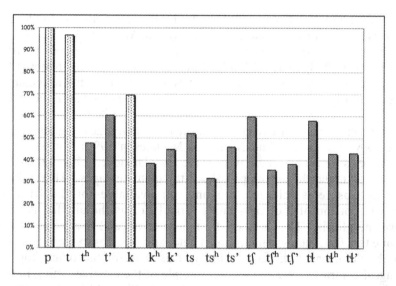

Figure 12 The ratio between the closure and the entire consonant duration (closure + release) of the Navajo stop series; the plain unapsirated stops (p, t, k), are lighter.

onsets that this characterization addresses is pertinent. Because the onsets of stems permit a complex set of articulations that are found nowhere else in the grammar, a straight phonemic analysis of the stops is slightly misleading. As we've noted, because of these constraints, it is difficult if not impossible to construct minimal pairs. The contrasts between the stop segments are realized primarily in the periods following the burst, the VOT's. Navajo makes ample use of this release period.

These stem onset articulations are characterized by whether or not the onset is simple or complex. If it's complex it has a closure period followed by a distinct release period. The release is a period in which laryngeal and manner contrasts are expressed. We can see this demonstrated in the spectrograms in Figure 13, of the prefix-noun tokens *bidił* [pɪtɪɬ], *bitoo'* [pɪtxʷoː'], *bit'iis* [pɪt'iːs], *bits'id* [pɪts'ɪt] and *bichiih* [pɪtʃʰiːh], for one female speaker. The plain coronal stop d [t] in *bidił* [pɪtɪɬ] is a simple onset. The others are complex onsets with distinct releases periods.

These spectrograms exemplify the profile of intervocalic stops, *d* [t] (176 ms), *t* [tx] (220 ms), *t'* [t'] (210 ms), *ts'* [ts'] (211 ms) and *ch* [tʃʰ] (201 ms) and the durations found in the chart in Figure 12. All but the unaspirated *d* [t] (first spectrogram in Figure 13), have a release period that is around 50% of the duration of the consonant, including the aspirated coronal stop *t* [tx] and, surprisingly, the ejectives. As discussed in McDonough and Ladefoged (1992) and first observed by Lindau (1984), the Navajo ejectives differ from ejectives found in other languages in the long period between the release of the oral gesture, indicated by the burst after the period of silence, and the release of the glottal gestures, indicated by the onset of the vowel formants. In our definition, this period is by definition the VOT. (See also the studies of ejectives on Western Apache (Southern Athabaskan) (Gordon et al. 2001) and on Witsuwit'en (Northern Athabaskan) (Wright at al. 2002) which found congruent patterns.) As McDonough and Ladefoged note, what is unusual about the articulation of these sounds is that this closure-release timing is maintained in the ejectives as well as the aspirated and affricated stops. Ejectives involve near simultaneous closure at two places in the oral cavity, at the glottis and at a place above the glottis (Ladefoged and Maddieson 1996). In Athabaskan, this oral closure is coronal, at or near the alveolar ridge. This oral closure is released first, and the air trapped above the glottis escapes. Thus, when the alveolar closure is released, the only air available for the fricated or aspirated portion of the consonant's articulation is the air that is trapped above the glottis. This is a small amount of air and it runs out quickly. Despite this fact, the glottal closure is held, and this closure period is around half the duration of the consonant, just as it is for the other stops with laryngeal contrasts. We can see an example of the ejective timing in the 3rd and 4th spectrograms in Figure 13, the tokens *bit'iis and bits'id*. Contrast the VOT of these ejectives, as I am defining it, with that of the aspirated stop *t* [tx] and affricate *ch* [tʃʰ] in the 2nd and 5th spectrograms. They are about equal. These two type consonants differ in the properties of their release periods. In the ejectives, the frication is narrow and ends well before the glottal release; in the aspirated and affricated stops, the release is fully fricated.

Contrast these four with the first spectrogram in Figure 13, the unaspirated coronal stop *d* [t]. This sound has no discernable VOT; the onset of voicing and vowel formants begins almost immediately after the release of the oral closure. Note also that a sharp onset of vowel formants and voicing is characteristic of all the stops, the unaspirated, aspirated and affricated series as well as the ejectives. The closure-release timing exemplified by these spectrograms is a striking characteristic of the stop series in Navajo. Considering all the duration measurements, it appears that the aspirated, affricated and ejective stops pattern together on the one hand and the unaspirated stops on the other. The aspirated, affricated and ejective stops have a long VOT of similar duration, while the unaspirated ones are very short. The VOT for all but the unaspirated stops makes up around half of the intervocalic stop consonant durations in the nouns in Navajo.

There is a relationship between the complexity of the onset and its duration; more complex onsets have longer durations than simple ones. That is, adding a gesture to the onset increases its length. We will see this further demonstrated in the discussion of the augmentative *x* (YM:gxiv) in Section 4.2.4.

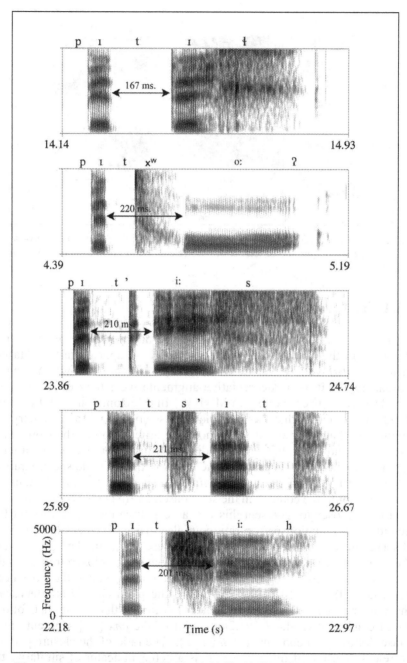

Figure 13 Spectrograms of *bidił, bitoo', bit'iis, bits'id* and *bichiih* demonstrating the stem-initial stop contrasts in intervocalic position. The windows are approximantly 780-880 ms in length.

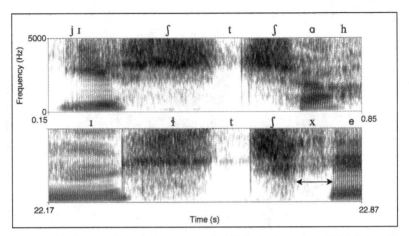

Figure 14 Characteristic spectrograms of *yishcha* (top), versus *ch'íniniłchxeeh*: one speaker. Note the differences in the release period of the stem's onset *ch* [tʃʰ].

4.2.4 The Augmentative

There is a morpheme which acts an augmentative or intensifier, appearing in the onset of the stems: the x [x]. It appears in the dataset in forms like *łitso* 'yellow' versus *łitsxo* 'orange' (intense yellow). Young and Morgan report it as a "depreciative-augmentative"; they describe it as a voiceless velar fricative [x] (YM:xiv). In McDonough and Ladefoged (1992), we reported that this morpheme *x* seemed to be a secondary type articulation that was carried throughout the articulation of the stop. In the current data, however, the *x* [x] is a distinct articulation that occurs after the stop, as we can see in the onset of the stems in the example spectrograms of *yishcha* (top) [jɪʃtʃʰɑh], versus *ch'íninilchxeeh* [tʃ'ɪn̩łtʃʰxe:h] in Figure 14. These exemplify the contrast in the stem onset: *ch* [tʃʰ] versus *chx* [tʃx].

I have chosen to represent this *x* as a velar fricative [x], as distinct from secondary articulation or aspiration in the affricate (see Chapter 5.3.4). Observe the closure to release ratio in these stops in the spectrograms. There are two conditioning factors that influence the closure/release ratios: whether the preceding segment is vowel or a consonant and the existence of the influx *x* [x]. In 13 of the 26 tokens, the plain *ch* [tʃʰ] is intervocalic. These intervocalic affricates are about 27% longer than those that follow a closed consonant (264.4 / 195.2ms). All of the *chx* [tʃx] segments in the dataset follow coda consonants (*sh* and *ł*). The ratio of the closure period to the release portion of the consonants is a better indicator of similarity than overall duration, i.e. the ratio of closure to release in the two environments is approximately the same independent of whether or not the consonant is preceded by a vowel or consonant.

The average duration of a *chx* [tʃx] is 218ms. The duration of the *chx* [tʃx] is more in keeping with the non-intervocalic (CC) *ch* [tʃʰ] (196ms) than with the VC environment (264ms). But the ratios of closure to release are different between the two type onsets, with and without the *x* [x]. The ratio of closure to release stands between .65 and .69 in the *ch* [tʃʰ] series (both CC and VC) (this includes what might be considered the aspiration). In the *chx* [tʃx] there are two measurements to consider: closure/release with and without the accompanying *x* [x]. The closure to release portion of the *chx* [tʃx] segment that does not include the accompanying *x* [x] is at .5; basically half closure and half release. The inclusion of the *x* [x] makes the release portion considerably longer and reduces the closure/release ratio to .32, which is quite low. This is exactly the inverse of the closure to release ratio of the *ch* [tʃʰ] tokens. Thus the accompanying *x* [x] seems to increase the duration of the release portion of the consonant. Since we have seen that the presence of a preceding consonant affects the durations of the following consonants, this may in effect be considered a sequence of a *ch* plus a *x*. I have written it as so. The inclusion of the *x* increases the duration of the onset.

This onset timing profile is also demonstrated in the waveforms for two pairs of the *litso* [ɬitsʰoh] 'yellow' / *litsxo* [ɬitsʰxoh] 'orange' contrast in two female speakers in Figure 15. The two tokens within each pair are approximately the same length. Note the consonant *ts* [tsʰ] is characterized by a closure period followed by a fricated release in all four tokens, but the 2nd and 4rd tokens also contain a distinct period of either weaker frication or aspiration after the affricate release, associated with the *x* [x] portion of the articulation. Note also that the more complex *tsx* onset is slightly longer than the *ts* in both speakers, in keeping with the general tendency for more complex onsets to be longer than simpler ones.

4.2.5 Verb Stem

Because of the verbal morphology, the distribution of verb stems is restricted to word-final position. As we have discussed, verbs are minimally bisyllabic due to the morphological imperative of the language; the verb is a compound of two syntactic domains. Thus verb stems are never found in word-initial position. In addition, because it is a compound boundary, the boundary between the two parts of the verb, Aux and Verb, is arguably different than the one between the prefix and the noun. We might expect to see this reflected in the phonetic implementation. In many instances, the prefixes to the noun were extremely short (McDonough and Ladefoged 1992); this is less the case with the pre-stem complex in verbs. Finally, because of the syllable shapes of the Aux stem (CV(V)(C)), the initial stop of the verb stem, then, can be found in either intervocalic position or preceded by a consonant depending on whether the Aux stem is open or

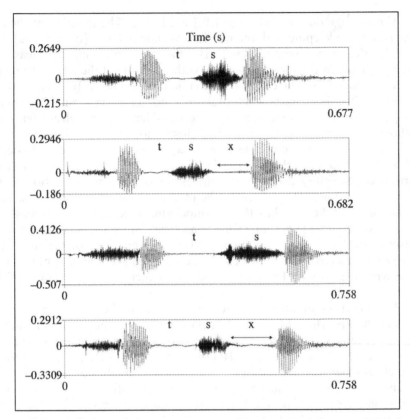

Figure 15 Two pairs of the litso/litsxo "yellow/orange" contrast: two female speakers.

closed. When an Aux stem has a coda, a consonant cluster appears in the word, and the verb stem is preceded by a consonant (..VC]+[CV..]). Example (1) demonstrates the two environments that the verb stem appears in: intervocalic or following a consonant.

(1)   VCV   VCCV
       yicha   yishcha
       [jɪ tʃʰɑh] [jɪʃ tʃʰɑh]

The possible codas that appear at the right edge of the penult syllable are the set of fricatives: *sh, s, ł, l*. In (1) we see the 1st and 3rd person singular forms of the ø-imperfective conjugation, *yish-* and *yi-* respectively. The verb stem is the imperfective form *cha* 'cry'.

Table 20 is a list of the durations of the stem onsets in the dataset. This dataset was not constructed to represent the full set of onset contrasts but to examine patterns within the verb. A comparison of the verb stem durations with the durations in Table 17 (whose median durations are repeated here as the final column of Table 20) shows that they are not dissimilar in duration, showing similar trends. As with the intervocalic noun stem consonants, the simple onsets in this dataset were shorter on average than the more complex ones. The glottal stop was the shortest onset, but the reliability of this duration figure is mitigated by the difficulty of accurately measuring the glottal stop due to the differences in its articulation across and within speakers. The *d* was shorter than the aspirated and ejective stops *t* and *t'*, but by a lesser degree than in the noun stems. And in fact the ejective *t'* is quite short by comparison to the nouns, almost 100 ms shorter (158.2 to 252.7) and it isn't much longer than the unaspirated *d* (153 ms) in this dataset.

Table 20 The consonant duration and distribution of the verb stem onsets as compared with the noun stems from Table 16 and Table 17(Navajo orthography).

YM	IPA	Median	St.Dev.	IQR	Count	Noun Stems
d	t	156.5	60.2	69.6	41	166.9
t	tx	183.3	32.2	46.4	27	230.5
t'	t'	158.2	40.5	45.7	25	252.7
k	kx	207.3	43.5	67.5	80	238.2
'	ʔ	97.4	29.1	46.9	42	
dz	ts	203.0	51.6	90.8	28	188.7
ts	tsʰ	225.0	73.3	70.6	13	210.3
ch	tʃʰ	213.4	55.8	72.7	26	235.4
chx	tʃʰx	218.0	42.7	40.6	26	
s	s	145.1	23.9	37.4	11	208.8
ł	ɬ	107.5	29.3	38.8	20	158.4
l	l	149.0	44.5	53.5	19	140.9
h	x	125.0	98.2	53.9	23	129.6
n	n	104.0	35.5	33.7	23	108
m	m	125.0	24.8	39.0	13	138.5

One significant factor that comes into play in the duration measurements of these verb onsets is the environment that they occur in. In the verb dataset under discussion, about 75% of the verb stems were in the consonantal environment, as opposed to the intervocalic environment of the noun stems. In the dataset, for instance, the ejective coronal stop *t'* appeared only in a consonantal environment. Table 21 is a chart of the verb stem consonants in intervocalic position.

We can see that the verb stem consonants tend on average to be longer than their noun counterparts. The nasal *m* has around the same duration and interquartile range (verb / noun) in both sets (124.6 / 138.5, IQR 39.2 / 28), as does the velar stop *k* (248.9 / 238.2, IQR 68.8 / 52.8) and to a lesser extent the affricates *ts* (254.4 / 210.3, IQR 71.7 / 14.7) and *ch* (265.2 / 235.4, IQR 50.9 / 21.7). But the voiced lateral *l* is quite different (249.4 / 140.9, IQR 52.9 / 70.6). However, because of the verbal morphology changes the

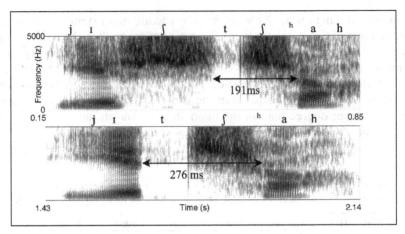

Figure 16 Characteristic spectrograms of *yishcha* (top), versus *yicha,* one speaker. Note the influence of the coda *sh* [ʃ] on the duration of the following affricate *ch* [tʃʰ].

status of the stem in the word, a comparison between these two sets of figures is difficult to evaluate.

Table 21 The duration for the verb stem initial consonants in an intervocalic position.

YM	IPA	Median	St.Dev.	Range	IQR	Count
ch	tʃʰ	265.2	42.3	168.6	50.9	14
dz	ts	254.4	56.2	180.4	71.7	14
m	m	124.6	24.8	72.2	39.2	13
k	kh	248.9	40.1	146.1	68.8	28
l	l	249.4	44.0	146.1	52.9	14
'	ʔ	96.0	33.2	126.1	50.2	22

Observe the example spectrograms of *yishcha* [jɪʃtʃʰah], versus *yicha* [jɪtʃʰah] for one female speaker in Figure 16. Each spectrogram window is approximately 705 ms in length. The closure / release of the intervocalic aspirated affricate *ch* [tʃʰ] in stem onset is 107/165 ms. The coda *sh* [ʃ] in *yishcha* is 216 ms long, and it has a discernable influence on the duration of the following onset (cl. 60 / rel.131). The intervocalic affricate is 85 ms longer than the one following the coda consonant *sh* [ʃ]. However in both cases, though the ratios of closure to release is slightly different in the two environments, it tends to follow the trend in VOT ratio's (*yishcha,* 0.45; *yicha,* 0.64).

Observe that for the 3rd person form *yicha* [jɪtʃʰah] the two syllables have the same shape (CV), despite the obvious differences in their duration. At first pass, this might be considered evidence for metric structure or foot-based phenomena. The first syllable is in a metrically weak position in the word, because the stem is prominent; therefore it is shorter. These type duration differences between strong and weak syllables are common. However, the 1st person form *yishcha* [jɪʃtʃʰɑh] doesn't share this effect. Its first syllable *yish-* [jɪʃ-] is quite long, due to the length of its coda. The shortness of the CV *yi* syllable cannot be argued to be a result of being in a weak position next to a prominent stem in a strong position, since this relationship does not apparently apply to the CVC syllable next to the stem. Instead I contend that evidence like this indicates that the duration differences between the stem and conjunct and disjunct domains are due to several incidental factors related to morphological and phonotactic structure. Little if any evidence can be found to support metric- or prosodic-based vowel or consonant duration effects. We will take up this discussion at the end of the chapter.

Note also that while both the closure and release period of the post-coda affricate is shorter, the closure period is more reduced than the release. These duration properties exemplified in the spectrograms illustrate properties of articulation of onsets found throughout the data. Also note that having a coda in the preceding syllable does not apparently affect the vowel of the stem syllable, as the vowel in both tokens is approximately the same, though the presence of a coda in a syllable does affect the duration of the syllable's vowel. Recall that the boundary between the stem and conjunct domain is the primary place in the word where consonant clusters may occur (see the discussion of the metathesis of *j-* in Chapter 3.7). The length of this final conjunct coda consonant, which is always a fricative, is a striking aspect of the conjunct domain, because when it is present, it is quite long. While the length of the stem codas can be attributed to their utterance-final position (the utterance being a single word in these cases), coda seems to be a position of lengthening, independent of whether they are utterance-final or not. We will return to this discussion in section 4.3.4.

Finally, if we consider the difference between simple and complex onsets, then the complex onsets in the verb dataset constituted more than half the onsets, 225 out of the 417 stem onsets. The simple onsets are the unaspirated plain stops, the glottal stop, and the continuants, the fricatives, nasals and glides. One question that arises with respect to the differences between the intervocalic onsets and those that follow a consonant is the closure-to-release ratio of stops in the verb dataset versus the nouns. Table 22 gives the closure-to-release ratios for the stop consonants in the verbs.

Note that the plain coronal stop *d* [t] has a very small release ratio. The velar stop *k* [kx], ejective *t'* [t'], the affricate *dz* [ts], are all around 50 % closure to release. The closure on the *t* [tx], and *ch* [tʃʰ] is smaller than half the duration of the consonant. The *ts* [tsʰ] has a very small closure period compared to its release. As mentioned many of these consonants follow a coda consonant, which tends to reduce the overall duration of the consonant and in particular its closure period.

Table 22 Closure-to-release ratios for stops in stems.

YM	IPA	Median	St.Dev.	Count
d	t	6.20	4.1	41
t	tx	0.55	0.2	27
t'	t'	0.91	0.7	25
k	kx	0.72	0.4	80
dz	ts	1.20	0.7	28
ts	tsʰ	0.36	0.3	13
ch	tʃʰ	0.67	0.3	52

The release periods of stops are an important aspect of the articulation and timing of consonants; they are not incidental gestures. In terms of the timing profile of the onset, both parts of the articulation of all but the unaspirated plain stops have a consistent duration and style that may be seen to indicate that these are complex onsets, that is to say, the phoneme inventory is an inventory of possible onsets.

4.3   CONJUNCT AND DISJUNCT DURATIONS

The conjunct and disjunct domains are domains of primarily prefixal morphemes. There are two sets of morphemes that are exceptions to this, the conjugational forms of the Base Paradigms (the Aux stems) and the Disjunct morphemes of position Ib, the so-called 'postpositional stems'. I have categorized the Base Paradigms (portmanteaus of Pos VII and VIII) as stems, for reasons discussed in Chapter 2, principally because these forms are the head of their domain (Auxiliary) and they exhibit the syllable shape and distribution of stems. However they differ from the noun and verb stems in exhibiting reduced contrasts, a characteristic of the prefixal morphemes of the Conjunct domain. The Disjunct postpositional stems of Ib have a larger set of contrasts (though not the full set), including affricates and ejectives, and vowel contrasts not normally found outside the verb and noun stems (ná- 'repitition', ch'í-' out horizontally', YM:g37), though they tend to have the prefixal CV syllable shape.

In this section we will examine the timing relationships among the consonants of the conjunct and disjunct domains. As before, I've reported the median, standard deviation and interquartile range (IQR) for all the consonant onsets. We will consider the conjunct consonants first.

4.3.1   The Conjunct Onset Consonants

Table 23 is a table of the stop consonants found in the conjunct domain in the dataset. I have excluded any consonant tokens (such as b [p]) that occur in initial position because of the difficulty of measuring these with any accuracy.

The coronal fricative *s* is the longest with a median of 154 ms, the glottal stop is the shortest with a median of 83 ms. This last figure is the least reliable, as many of the glottal stops in the language vary freely with creaky voice, which is difficult to measure with any accuracy. (The reported measurements were made of the clear closure period in the articulation of the glottal stop, and do not include the vocal fold striations of creaky voice, that is to say measurements were taken of the glottal stops as complete stops, and not as a phonation type.) Apart from the nasal *n* which we will consider in the next section (4.3.2), the *d* [t] is the most common segment in the dataset.

Table 23 Conjunct onsets durations in word-medial position in ms.

YM	IPA	Median	Std.Dev.	IQR	Count
h	x	92.25	35.157	43.8	46
s	s	154.2	20.314	22.35	8
d	t	123.55	41.015	43.65	196
'	ʔ	83	49.341	82.95	24

It is difficult, as we have noted, to compare the consonants in the stem and conjunct domains because of the differences in the distribution of the phonemic contrasts between the two domains. All manner and laryngeal contrasts and most of the place of articulation contrasts are absent. The differences between the consonants in stem onset and in the conjunct domain can be demonstrated by examining an instance of a non-initial conjunct consonant, the unaspirated coronal stop *d* [t].

Measurements were made of both the closure duration and the release duration of this stop as a point of comparison with the stem-initial *d* [t]. As with all the unaspirated stops, the VOT of the conjunct *d* is quite small. Recall that VOT is measured from the release of the oral closure to the onset of voicing in the vowel. A spectrogram of the *d* [t] conjunct onset and stem-initial position for two speakers is shown in Figure 17.

This spectrogram exemplifies several aspects of the timing properties in the verb. Note the characteristic pattern in the initial ejective affricate *ch'* [tʃ'], 'out horizontally' at the disjunct domain (section 4.2.2); this is a morpheme from position Ib. Also note the length contrast between the two lateral fricatives, both in coda position, the voiced approximant lateral at the edge of the conjunct domain (171 / 131 ms) versus the voiceless final lateral fricative (348 / 352 ms). Relevant to the present discussion, note the two *d*-[t] segments, in conjunct and stem initial position (128 / 184 ms, top spectrogram, 69 / 90 ms, bottom). These are marked by arrows in the spectrograms. The VOT on the *d* [t] consonants in both conjunct and stem initial position is not much larger than the release burst, we can see this in the spectrograms in Figure 17.

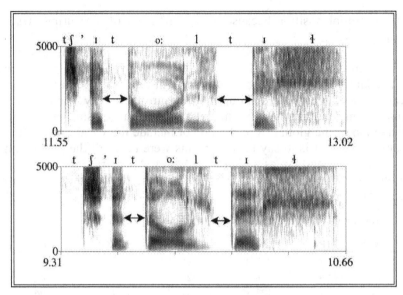

Figure 17 Characteristic spectrograms of *ch'ídooldił* [tʃ'ɪtoːltɪɬ]: two female speakers. Arrows indicate the duration of the plain unaspirated stop *d* [t].

The median and standard deviation for the *d* segment in the conjunct domain is 123.55 (41) ms. The interquartile range is 43.65 ms. The conjunct *d* [t] was present in 14 out of 32 of the verbs. Compare these figures to the stem *d*, where the median (standard deviation) is 156 (61) ms, and IQR is 73.2 Thus the median, standard deviation and range of the stem onset was larger than that of the conjunct *d* [t]. The stem initial *d* is 21% longer than the conjunct *d*. In addition, in the dataset, the stem initial consonant *d* is not in intervocalic position, as the conjunct consonant is. As we've seen, the stem consonants that follow a coda (CC-type) are on average shorter than the intervocalic stem consonants.

Table 24 Stem vs. conjunct durations for d, h, and s.

	Median	s.d.	IQR	count
Stem d	156	61	73.2	40
Conj d	123.6	41	43.7	196
Stem h	125	98.2	53.9	23
Conj h	92.3	32	43.8	46
Stem s	145	23.5	37.3	11
Conj s	154.2	20.3	23.4	8

The same pattern holds true of the *h*- segment, the aspirated glottal fricative. In stem initial position in the verb, the median, standard deviation and IRQ s are 125 (98.2), 53.9 over 23 tokens; in the conjunct domain: 92.3 (32), 43.8 over 46 tokens. The stem-initial *h* is 27% longer than the *h* in conjunct. Again the stem-initial *h* is not in intervocalic position. The alveolar fricative *s* segment does not follow the same pattern, for if we compare the verb stem to the conjunct, we see that the conjunct s is slightly longer; however there is a large difference between the noun (208 ms) and verb stems figures for s, and a comparison of the noun to conjunct durations, the noun stem s is 26% longer than the conjunct.

4.3.2   Conjunct Nasals

The nasals presented a particular problem to the analysis of segment durations and we will consider them separately. The coronal stop d [t] and the coronal nasal *n* are by far the most common consonants in the conjunct domain accounting for nearly 83% of all the consonantal onsets in the dataset, and the nasals are slightly more common (by count, nasal, 247; d, 196 of the 512 conjunct onsets). While the conjunct domain syllables are CV, when a nasal was present in the conjunct domain, some speakers produce it as a syllabic nasal (*ni* → n). Navajo has these two distinct patterns: a nasal consonant articulation with a clear onset and offset followed by a vowel articulation, and a realization of the syllable as a syllabic nasal. Figure 18 illustrates this. The disjunct- conjunct sequence *ch'íninil-* from the word *ch'íninilkaad,* uttered by two female speakers, is illustrated in the spectrogram.

The spectrograms illustrate variations in the articulation of nasal + vowel sequences. The top and middle spectrograms are two tokens of the utterance *ch'ininishkaad,* [tʃ'mmʃkxaat] from two different speakers. The bottom spectrogram is from a token of the word *ch'ininilchxeeh* [tʃ'mɬtʃʰxeeh]. The middle and bottom spectrograms are from the same speaker. Note the variation in the articulation of the nasal +vowel sequence across these three utterances. In the top spectrogram, the speaker pronounced both syllables as a clear nasal+vowel sequence [-nɪnɪ-] (the second nasal + vowel sequence is 200ms long (nasal 123ms, *i,* 76 ms)) In the middle spectrogram, the sequence *-nini-* is pronounced as a nasal +vowel + syllabic nasal [-nɪn̩] (the syllabic nasal is 260 ms long). In the bottom spectrogram, this same speaker pronounced a long syllabic nasal [-n̩-] (360ms) in place of the (orthographic) *-nini-.* Note also that these variations occur both across and within speakers.

In this dataset, the nasal + vowel was more common than the syllabic nasal, arguably due to the careful speech style of the data collection, although a couple of speakers tended to produce long syllabic nasals (in particular, the two male speakers, who had a more casual style speech)[6]. This alternation is worthy of mention because the syllabic nasal is not an allophone of a nasal + vowel sequence in stem onsets; it only occurs in the disjunct and conjunct domains.

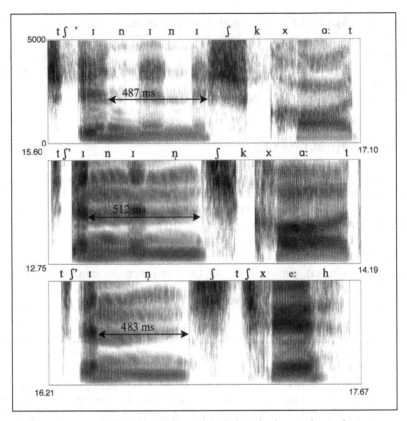

Figure 18 Spectrograms illustrating the variations in the nasal-vowel sequences in *ch'íninish-* [tʃ'ɪnɪnɪʃ] from *ch'ininishkaad* and *ch'ininishchééh*: two female speakers.

This variability in the articulation of nasal syllables is reflected in the domain durations (section 4.1). In the dataset wordlists, there were 8 verbs with conjunct domains that consisted of nasal sequences. Half of these were one syllable long and the other half were two syllables long.

If we consider the duration of a nasal syllable in these two-syllable conjunct domains to be 1/2 the duration of the whole domain then the syllables in two syllable conjunct domains are 262ms., versus 307 in a monosyllabic conjunct, as shown in Table 25. Again, because the data set was not set up to examine this phenomena, comparisons of this type are best taken as patterns in the data that indicate the need for closer study of a phenomenon. However, the comparison is useful in describing an observable pattern; the difference in duration between a nasal syllable in a one-syllable versus two-syllable domain is 58.2ms, the difference in the IQR is 105.3ms. If the nasals were the same duration in both 1- and 2- syllable conjunct domains, we'd expect the differences in the duration of a nasal syllable between the two domains to average around 0, with a small standard deviation, and a narrow interquartile range. But the mean is not centered around 0. The differences between the two groups of nasal syllables centers well above 0, and the standard deviation is large. It appears that nasal syllables in one-syllable domains have a tendency to be longer than those in two-syllable domains on the whole, and their IQR's are smaller. There is a great deal of speaker variability but the variability errs on the side of longer monosyllabic conjunct nasals, although the data show that this difference is not statistically significant in this dataset.

Table 25 Durations of two- and one- syllable conjunct domain consisting of nasal + vowel or syllabic nasal sequences.

	Count	Median (perσ)	St.Dev.	Range	IQR
1σ	14	524	138.9	461.5	153
2σ	14	307	82.6	344.7	59

Also note that the 2-syllable conjunct domains all had codas, while only half the one-syllable conjuncts did. Since codas make the syllable longer, and are associated with longer domains, this distribution fact biases the data in the direction of longer durations for two-syllable conjunct nasals.

Thus, in keeping with the general tendency of the conjunct domain characterized by the syllable score (section 4.1), doubling the numbers of syllables in a domain does not double the length of the domain. The question that remains to be discovered is the exact nature of this phenomenon. An analysis of weak / strong syllable pattern is very difficult to construe given the facts we see here. The stem syllable is arguably the strongest in the word. An alternating metric pattern would make the adjacent syllable, the penult syllable, weak. This is not consistently the case. Syllable duration seems to depend on a variety of factors, including segment type and domain length. The fact that nasal consonants are in such a large number of conjunct syllables, that these can be compressed into what are apparently shorter syllabic nasals, or that two-syllable conjunct domains are have a mean syllable duration that is shorter than the one-syllable domains means that if a weak / strong pattern is in effect, it is qualified by a large enough number of segmental and timing factors to make a metric analysis at best problematical.

4.3.3 Conjunct Glides

There were several examples of glide-vowel conjunct domains (*yi-* and *yish-*). Stevens (2002) has pointed out that the acoustic discontinuties associated with glide vowel sequences are weak or not present at all, which holds true of the Navajo data, making segmentation of the glide vowel sequence arbitrary. We can see this in the spectrogram of a glide-vowel-glide-vowel conjunct sequence, *yiyii* [jɪjɪː] from the verb *yiyiisxį* in Figure 19.

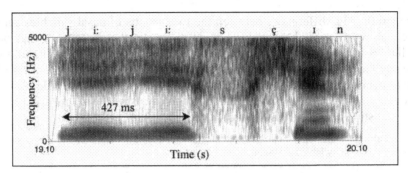

Figure 19 Spectrogram for *yiyiisxị̇*, demonstrating a characteristic pattern of glide-vowel sequences.

Other examples of *yi* or *yish* sequences can be found in the spectrograms in Figure 16 and Figure 20. Segmentation of the glide vowel sequence is too arbitrary for an accurate measurement of duration for the individual segments.

4.3.4 Codas in the Stem and Conjunct Domains

The averages, standard deviations and count for the coda consonants in the conjunct domain by segment are shown in Table 26. There are 309 codas in the conjunct domain in this dataset, and all of these, except the *zh* (8 by count) are in the coda of a syllable at the right edge of a domain; either the final syllable in the word or the penult syllable (the edge of the conjunct domain), as shown by the underlined segments in (2).

(2)   [(…) [CVV<u>C</u>]stem]Aux [[CVV<u>C</u>] stem]Verb

The single place in the word where a consonant cluster consistently appears is between the last two syllables in the verb word, due to the concatenation of an Aux stem with a coda (i.e. *yish-* øimp/1s) and the consonant initial verb stem. An example is *yishcha* [jɪʃtʃʰah] (spectrogram in Figure 16), the Aux stem is the ø imperfective/ 1ˢᵗ singular *(y)ish-* [jɪʃ], resulting in a consonant cluster –ʃtʃʰ- at the conjunct stem boundary.

The *zh* [ʒ], italicized in the data Table 26, is the only coda that is not in domain final position. Other than the syllable that contains this segment, the syllables of the conjunct Infl domain (outside the Base Paradigms) are open (CV). This segment *zh* represents a unique morpheme, the 'deictic subject' marker for 3ʳᵈ impersonal; it has unique distribution pattern in that it appears to metathesize (CV→VC) (Section 3.7). In this dataset, this morpheme *ji-* (*dzi-* by harmony), has metathesized to a coda position, as in *bik'ihozhdii'ą́'* 'you blame him'[7]. This is the single instance of a conjunct-internal coda.

Table 26 Conjunct domain coda consonant durations.

YM	IPA	Median	St.Dev.	Range	IQR	Count
h	h	43.7	40.8	118.0	28.1	6
s	s	194.9	44.7	169.3	67.2	27
sh	ʃ	189.2	43.5	239.6	58.1	209
z	z	112.6	52.7	124.6	64.3	4
ł	ɬ	147.8	37.6	127.7	59.8	25
l	l	137.1	35.5	179.6	35.2	27
zh	ʒ	123.2	19.6	57.0	31.0	8
Overall		176.7	51.1	318.9	66.4	309

Outside this conjunct-internal coda morpheme, there are 318 codas in this dataset, out of a possible 448 coda positions (32 words x 14 speakers). The most frequent coda is the voiceless palato-alvealor fricative *sh* [ʃ], which also has the longest duration, followed in frequency by the voiceless alvealor fricative *s*. The voiced and voiceless laterals do not differ significantly in length. Both the *s* and the *sh* occur as the coda in the Base Paradigms. The *sh* is the morphome (in the sense of Aronoff 1992), or the functor, for 1st subject. It may appear as *s* under harmony due to the presence of an alveolar fricative in the verb stem. The *s* may also indicate the 3rd singular form in some conjugational paradigms (see the Base Paradigm chart in YM (g200-1). The lateral fricatives are the "classifiers' or valence markers to the verb stem, as part of the Verb constituent. These morphemes appear in this position, domain final, via a prosodic process that incorporates them into this coda position when it is open to them; i.e. when the form from a Mode paradigm is an open syllable (CV/ CVV, such as the 2nd sing, n-imperfective *ni*). This is part of a more general prosodic process which bars the affixes to the verb stem from appearing as affixes; basically it bars any material from breaking the alignment of the boundary of the stem to the boundary of the syntactic domain Verb, and it causes a series of phonological and prosodic effects, such as inducing mutation on the initial consonant of the verb stem (as in the d-effects and voicing reflex of fricatives in onset of the verb stem) (Section 3.6.1). Of interest to us here is the duration weight that the final consonant brings to the size of the conjunct domain. We can see this phenomena in the spectrograms of *yishcha* [jɪʃtʃʰɑh], versus *yicha* [jɪtʃʰɑh], from one female speaker in Figure 16.

Each spectrogram is approximately 705 ms in length. The coda *sh* is 216 ms long, and it has a discernable influence on the duration of the following onset, which is the aspirated affricate *ch* [tʃʰ]. The intervocalic affricate is 85 ms longer than the one following the coda consonant *sh*. Note also in this spectrogram that while both the closure and release period of the post-coda affricate have been reduced, the closure period is more reduced than the release. These duration properties exemplified in the spectrograms represent trends found throughout the data. Also note that

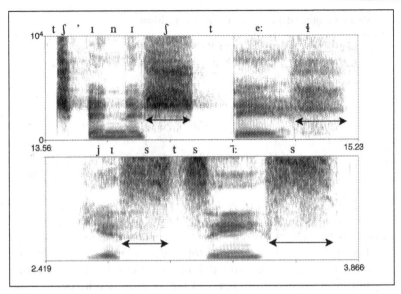

Figure 20 Spectrograms of *ch'ínishdeeł* [tʃʼınıʃteːɬ] and yisdzį́į́s [jıstsĩːs], from the same speaker. Note the length of the coda consonants (arrows).

having a coda in the preceding syllable does not apparently affect the vowel of the stem syllable, the vowel in both tokens is approximately the same, though the presence of a coda in a syllable does affect the duration of the vowel in that syllable. The length of this final coda consonant, which is always a fricative (s, ʃ, ɬ, l, h), is a striking aspect of the conjunct domain. When a coda is present, it is distinctly long. This comes into play in a discussion of the stem codas, which can also be quite long. While the length of the stem codas can be attributed to their position as final in the utterance (which is a single word in these cases), coda position in general seems to be a position of lengthening, independent of whether they are utterance final or not.

It was possible to measure the durations of many of the word final coda consonants because it was possible to establish where the consonant ended in most cases. We can see this demonstrated in Figure 20, which contains spectrograms of *ch'ínishdeeł* [tʃʼmıʃteːɬ] (top) and yisdzį́į́s [jıtsĩːs] (bottom) from the same speaker. In both spectrograms, there is a consonant cluster at the conjunct / stem juncture, (-*shd*- [-ʃt-] and -*sdz*- [-sts-], respectively), which is between the penult and final syllable.

Note the length of the two codas in each spectrogram (marked by arrows). Because of consonant harmony, the conjunct coda must harmonize to the stem, removing anteriority contrasts between the conjunct coda and the stem. This is apparent in the bottom spectrogram, where the *yish* (øimp/1s) appears as *yis*- [jıs-] due to the presence of the [+anterior] stem *dzį́į́s*.[tsĩːs] (Chapter 3). Note the articulation of the two affricates, the ejective affricate *ch'* [tʃʼ] in the top spectrogram, with its characteristic ejective VOT (section 4.2.1), and the stem-initial affricate *dz* [ts] in the bottom spectrogram, discussed in section 4.2.5. Observe the stem initial *d* [t] segment in the top spectrogram, with its very short, burst sized, VOT and its sharply delineated offset. Note also the quality of the vowel formants and the vowel-nasal-vowel sequence in the top spectrogram, where the nasal is quite clearly articulated. All these are characteristics of the Navajo speech in this dataset.

As we can see in Table 27, the stems codas are quite long. As with the conjunct codas, the fricatives are the longest, the glottal aspirate *h* is the shortest. Unlike the other fricatives, the glottal fricative was somewhat difficult to measure because there was no clear offset to its articulation, as Figure 20 demonstrates. The *d* coda segments were measured at their release.

Table 27 Stem coda durations.

IPA	Median	St.Dev.	Range	IQR	Count
d	91.4	56.9	267.6	64.0	75
h	74.9	44.0	237.6	59.3	162
l	226.5	92.8	359.2	138.7	45
s	299.7	78.2	400.1	103.5	51
ʃ	241.5	86.0	326.6	133.8	21
z	253.8	87.4	216.5	158.7	6
Overall	116.6	107.0	475.3	155.7	380

Not surprisingly, given what we have seen in the conjunct codas, the codas in word-final position are also long, and they are longer than the conjunct codas. The stem codas are statistically very distinct from the conjunct codas (t (308) = -3.59, p < .0004). This feature is a probable result of final lengthening, a common effect of segmental lengthening that occurs at the edges of an utterance. The stem codas are in word final position and the words were said in isolation. However, this same citation production makes it impossible to determine the nature of any final lengthening effect in this data. As noted above, the conjunct codas are also quite long, so the length of the codas cannot be due entirely to their position at the right edge of an utterance since the conjunct codas are internal to the word, though they are at the right edge of their domain. However, as we can see in the spectrograms throughout this chapter, this edge between the conjunct and stem (the penult and ultimate syllable), a point where the two domains meet, is an outstanding characteristic in the acoustic profile of the verb word.

4.3.5 Disjunct Domain Durations

Of the 32 words in the dataset, 21 of them had a disjunct domain, and stops were in initial position in 18 of the 21 disjunct words. As such the

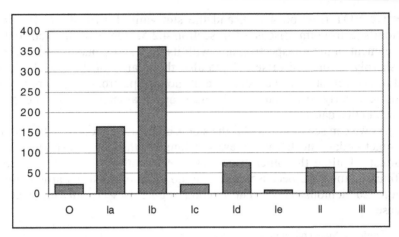

Figure 21 The disjunct domain morpheme frequencies in Young and Morgan (1987) by position (from Sussman and McDonough 2002).

measurements of the closure period of stops were difficult to make with any accuracy, so care should be taken when comparing the figures for these onsets to either the stems or to non-initial conjunct consonants. The figures for the stops *ch', dz* and *k'* are of their release periods alone, and as such they are comparable to the release periods of other stops, since the differences are not statistically significant.

Examples of an initial disjunct prefix is found in Figure 20; the top half of the figure is a spectrogram of the word *ch'ínishdeeł* [tʃ'ınıʃte:ɬ]. All of the disjunct prefixes in the dataset belong to Position Ib, the position of the postpositional stems. These morphemes exhibit a larger set of contrasts than do the other prefixes; there are affricates and ejectives in this Ib group, their syllable shape is principally CV or CVV, as we can see from the template morpheme list in YM (g37). In Figure 21 are the counts for the morphemes in the disjunct domain by position. The figures were calculated over the dictionary entries in Young and Morgan (1987)[8], since frequencies of production in actual speech were unavailable.

Table 28 Disjunct onset consonant durations.

YM	Median	St.Dev.	IQR	Count
h	121.1	37.669	37.4	18
n	104.9	63.514	56.575	47
ch'	136.6	39.096	61.225	123
dz	134.25	44.251	72.9	26
k'	212.5	113.911	183	62

Among the entries in the Young and Morgan dictionary, these Ib postpositional morphemes are the most commonly occurring morpheme in the disjunct domain. This indicates that their relative phonotactic prominence and frequency is likely to have a defining influence on the profile of this domain. Since the more complex segments are longer than the simple segments, and since the Ib consonants in the dataset are not statistically distinct in duration from the stem consonants, the frequency of the Ib morphemes are a likely cause of the differences between the disjunct and conjunct syllable scores in Section 4.1. That is to say, the differences between the disjunct and conjunct domain duration patterns are likely to be a result of the combination of gross phonotactic structure constraints, and their timing footprints, and morpheme frequency patterns, rather than any higher level phenomena such as any properties inherent to organization of syllables or to the domains or the morphemes themselves.

4.4   VOWEL LENGTH BY DOMAIN

In this section the duration measurements of the vowels in the word are described. In particular we are interested in the length contrast and in the differences between the long and short vowels of the stem versus conjunct and disjunct domains.

4.4.1   The Duration of Vowels in Navajo

The durations of the long and short vowels in the noun and verb data are listed in the following tables. Note that the long vowels are more than twice the length of the short vowels. The largest difference between long and short vowels is in the noun stems, the noun measurements are of isolated disyllabic (prefix + noun) tokens.

As can be seen from the data in Table 29, Navajo speakers make very clear distinctions between long and short vowels, at least when producing citation forms. Short vowels were less than half the length of long vowels. The difference between long and short vowels in each domain was statistically significant (Verb stems, t (9) = -6.9, p<.0001; Conjunct, t (116) = -15.2, p<.0001; Disjunct, t (9) = -6.9, p<.0001; Noun stems t (116) = -20.3, p<.0001). These duration measurements represent true contrasts between long and short vowels within a stem. The length contrast can be considered a very robust contrast in Navajo. The difference between the long vowels, but not the short vowels, in the stem domains versus the conjunct domains is also statistically significant (t (114) =-11.1 , p<.0001). Thus there is a difference between the long versus short vowels in the dataset. This difference is demonstrated in Figure 22.

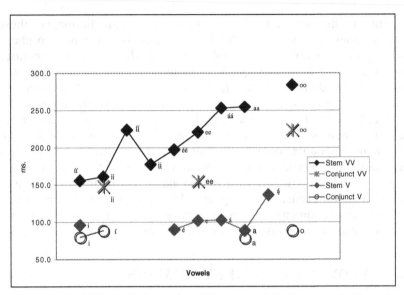

Figure 22 The long and short vowels in the verb, by domain (Navajo orthography).

We can see that for each vowel quality with the exception of the long high front vowel *ii*, there are larger differences in the long versus the short vowels between the conjunct (circles and stars) and stem (solid squares and triangles) domains. The short vowels are more similar to each other in duration. It is also important to recall the strong distribution constraints at work in these domains, reflected in the distribution counts in Table 30.

Table 29 Vowel duration medians. standard deviations and IQR's in milliseconds of nouns and verbs.

	Median	St.Dev.	IQR	Count
Stem				
V	97.8	48.543	41	114
VV	218.85	65.308	86.05	288
Conjunct				
V	77.1	29.283	32.475	435
VV	147.2	45.014	60	116
Disjunct				
V	76.55	37.241	36.25	276
VV	182.2	22.786	37.425	9
Noun Stem				
V	94.1	56.217	62.5	278
VV	250.9	84.095	104.3	234

As we can see from Table 29 there are differences between the long stem and conjunct vowels, but the short vowels are more similar in duration.

There are a few things to keep in mind. First, there is no symmetry in the distribution of vowel contrasts in either quality, length, nasality or tone, as we can see from the gaps in the table. In this dataset, there are 111 short vowels in the stem, compared to 431 in the conjunct domain. This means that there are almost 4 times as many short vowels in the conjunct than the stem domain. In the conjunct domain, the short vowels are primarily the high front vowel *i* (362 out of 431 vowels), as expected, given the default status of many of the vowels in this domain. The round vowels are associated with the *ho-* 3rd (animate / space) Agr prefix group and optative conjugation. The low vowels are associated with the *'a-* 3rd ('someone/thing unspecified') Agr prefix group.

Table 30 The distribution counts for the long and short vowels by domain and category in the dataset (Navajo orthography).

VV	stem	conjunct	V	stem	conjunct
íí	24		i	25	156
ii	6	90	í		206
į́į́	36				
įį	15				
éé	39		é	25	
ee	26	12	e	2	
áá	41		á	16	
aa	39		a	23	22
			ą	20	
oo	13	13	o		47
Total	239	115	Total	111	431
		Grand Total		350	546
				Stem	Conj

As we can see, the conjunct domain has half as many long vowels as the stem (Stem = 239, Conjunct =115). Recall that the long vowels in the pre-stem prefix complex are either from the Aux stem, the disjunct domain or they are derived over the disjunct / conjunct boundary. The figures in these charts and tables consider only underived long vowels, that is to say that the long conjunct vowels are those of the Aux stems. The long round vowel *oo* appeared in only one verb stem, *bidiniiltsood,* the conjunct long vowel appeared in the verb *ch'ídooldeeł* (see Appendix I for the wordlists in this study), in the optative conjugation (Aux stem, *oo(h)* opt/2nd d). Long vowels that were composed of morphemes from the disjunct and conjunct domains (*ch'óóshdeeł* → *ch'í # [ósh] [ł-deeł]*)[9] were not considered in this count, although long vowels that arose from morpheme combinations within the conjunct were counted (*'aniishháásh* → *'(a)-n(i)-(y)i-ish-háásh*). (Recall in the algorithm used in this study, the prefixes from Qu and Agr groups are attached to the Aux stem, YM's Base Paradigms. As such the forms of the Aux stem are not constructed via concatenation and the long vowels in these paradigms are underlying.). High front nasal conjunct vowels were not counted because of the tendency for *n+i* sequences to become syllabic nasals. All the long vowels in the disjunct domain come from one morpheme, *náá*. The short vowels were primarily *i* (229/277), as expected. The disjunct prefix vowel durations are similar to the conjunct vowel durations. Nearly all of the disjunct morphemes are Ib morphemes (18/21).

In the stems, the vowel qualities were more evenly distributed, though this dataset was not constructed to control for vowel quality distribution; there is no information on phoneme frequencies available as yet on Navajo. There were no statistically significant differences between any of the vowel qualities within a vowel length (long or short) within a domain. Given the asymmetries between the distribution of vowel qualities among the domains, this fact makes comparison of vowel durations between the different domains reasonable.

Because of the significant differences between the durations of long and short vowels, and because significant differences extend across the conjunct and stem domains for the long but not short vowels, an account of the duration differences between the stem and conjunct domains as a result of the prosody of final lengthening is weakened. If the duration of the vowels in the stem domain was influenced by final lengthening, we'd expect similar effects on both the long and the short vowels, that is to say both the long and short vowels would show statistically significant differences between the stem domain and the conjunct domain. But we do not find statistically significant differences between the short vowels in any of the domains; the short vowels are similar in duration across domains. It appears that long vowels in the stems have a tendency to be longer than those in pre-stem complex while on the whole, short vowels do not. The nature of this difference is unclear, but it is perhaps related to the fact that long vowels are uncommon outside the stem domain and short vowels are uncommon within it.

Finally note the differences in the duration of the short vowels and the consonants in the conjunct domain. The consonants are longer than the vowels by about 35 ms on average, and the difference is statistically significant (t (292) = 14.1, p<.0001). Thus the conjunct domain is a domain of primarily CV syllables, whose onsets are longer then the nuclei, with a long domain-final coda.

4.5   STRESS IN THE VERB

The stem domain is a domain of long vowels, codas, contrasts and complex onsets. The conjunct domain is a domain of reduced contrasts, CV syllables with short nuclei and simple onsets. Insofar as this is the case, these distribution facts alone may account in large part for the distinct durational profiles of the two domains captured by the syllable score figure.

There is presently no way of checking the distributional frequencies of the shapes of the conjunct and stem domains in verbs in the Navajo lexicon; however a check through the root and stem dictionary (Appendix V, g318-356) and the list of conjunct prefixes (g37-38) in YM tends to substantiate this observation. A further check for morpheme distribution tendencies in a 15,000 word database drawn from a digitalized version of the Young and Morgan dictionary (the 1999 Lockard CD of the Young and Morgan 1987 volume) indicates that of the total entries, most consist of a Base Paradigm form (Aux stem) and classifier + verb stem, that is to say, the bisyllabic core verb ([Aux]+[Verb]). Outside the core verb, the most common morphemes that appear in the dictionary are the conjunct Pos. V 'deictic subject' (Agr) morphemes, and the disjunct Pos. Ib, the postpositional stems. While these distributional facts reflect the entries in a dictionary, that is to say, they reflect the structure of the dictionary and may not reflect word usage or actual morpheme frequency, the dictionary indicates that a large number of Navajo verbs are likely to be short (given the complexity of the morphology). Willie (pc) has made a similar observation. The duration and timing facts laid out in this chapter indicate that shorter verb words will tend to lend prominence to stems based on phonotactics and syllable structure asymmetries alone.

If we factor away from the durational effects of phonotactic asymmetries, very little is left in the way of evidence for the presence of structurally encoded phenomena like stress, accent or metric structure as an explanation of the timing and duration facts in Navajo. The metric and prosodic structure that a particular language within the family has developed, may be the most likely, and the most systematic, way in which the Athabaskan languages differ from one another. I suggest that research into this area is likely to yield significant results in many important areas of Athabaskan studies.

We have seen that the differences between the disjunct and conjunct domains may well lie in the kinds of morphemes that are showing up with the greatest frequency in the disjunct domain, i.e. the postpositional stems and their enlarged contrasts (relative to the inflectional domains). I suggest that this is also true of the difference between the profiles of the stem versus conjunct domains. The stems have the contrasts, which includes the consonantal contrasts and long vowels, tone, nasality and the four vowel qualities, whereas these contrasts are present in the prefix complex either not at all or as marked or contextual features.

If particular prosodic structures, like stress or metric structure, were present in the verb, we would expect to see a consistent expression of features related to stress, such as duration, timing and vowel quality differences that have been found in languages with stress and metric systems. We do not find this. Instead the principal indications of the duration of the conjunct domain are the presence of codas, the number of syllables and the presence of long vowels. Codas do not occur freely; they are morphologically constrained arguably to right edges of domains. The greatest indication of a syllable's length in both the conjunct and stem domain is whether or not it has a coda, not its position relative to a strong syllable (section 4.3.4).

The last syllable in the word, the verb stem, is a content morpheme. Because the language is verb final it is also likely to be the last word in a larger domain of reference, such as a sentence (syntactic) or utterance (prosodic) level. This syllable is prominent on many levels. But little, if any, evidence can be construed from the data in this chapter for the straightforward play of metric or prosodic structure above the syllable level in the grammar of Navajo. This is not to say that it does not exist. But if it does, it is not apparently obvious in the timing and duration facts of the verb.

4.6 OVERVIEW OF DURATION FACTORS AND THE NAVAJO VERB

Rigid morpheme ordering and constraints on the distribution of contrasts means that featural contrasts occur in a single highly constrained position in the word, in the last syllable of the verb, its right edge, which has the morphological status of stem in the grammar (Section 2.6). Stems are morphemes of complex onsets, vowels contrasts, long vowels and codas. The pre-stem domains, disjunct and conjunct, are domains of primarily CV syllables and reduced contrasts. In a system like this, the notion 'minimal pair' as a way of determining (and, presumably, learning (Maye 2002)) contrasts, is not entirely functional. The phonemic inventory of Navajo in Table 9, and by extension of Athabaskan, is basically a list of the possible onsets in stems. The contrasts in onsets move from simple articulatory gestures, like those found in fricatives and simple approximants, to more elaborate gestures like affricates, and to complex gestures such as aspirated lateral affricates and ejectives; also, the onsets tend to increase in size across the groups as they gain in complexity (sections 0 and 0). This last feature is tied to the fact that the stem onsets are characterized by a consistent timing footprint which tends to preserve or enhance the release portions of stops series. It is in this release portion, which I have called VOT for expository purposes, that the contrasts of the more complex segments are realized. These contrasts are thus necessarily manner and laryngeal contrasts and not place contrasts, since release periods, cross-linguistically, are unlikely locations for place contrasts to be realized (heterorganic affricates are rare, for instance). Consilient to this is a harmony process in Navajo which bars the core verb, at least, from exhibiting anteriority (place) contrasts among the strident fricatives (Chapter 3.3).

The conjunct and disjunct domains, with the exception of Pos. Ib, the postpositional stems, are the domains of simple segments, that is simple articulatory gestures like the unaspirated coronal stop and the approximants, with few place contrasts. These domains are arguably domains of primarily inflectional morphemes, and cross-linguistically inflectional morphemes tend to be comprised of segments that are articulatorily simple, unmarked gestures in the sense of Lindblom and Maddieson (1989). In addition, the consonants in CV syllables in the Navajo verb, across the domains, tend to be longer than the (short) vowels in these syllables. This means that the conjunct domain tends to have a stronger consonantal profile, contrasted with the stem and, to a lesser degree, the disjunct domains.

The juncture between the stem and conjunct domains is a prominent place in the word, as we can see from the spectrograms in this chapter. It is the single place where a consonant cluster occurs, due to the presence of a domain final coda in the conjunct domain (Chapter3). Codas in general are quite long; the stem codas are longer than the conjunct (section 4.3.4), possibly due to the prosodic effects such as final lengthening, which is known to lengthen segments that occur at the edges of domains in English. Being preceded by a coda reduces the duration of a stem-initial onset, affecting closure period more than the release. This is demonstrated in spectrograms such as Figure 14.

Finally, the stems are prominent in the word, though this prominence is complex and it is not obviously due to timing relationship between syllables that can be argued to be governed by higher level prosodic phenomena such as foot structure. Instead the prominence seems to be governed by the inherent asymmetries in the phonotactics of each domain and the category of a morpheme.

In the next chapter we turn to the spectral characteristics of the sounds.

---

[1] The verb stem and the classifier (= the verb base) constitute the Verb domain in the bipartite view. However, due to the phonology of the classifier prefixes, the Verb domain is always a single syllable and is congruent to the verb stem (Chapter 3.6.1). The classifier never appears as a CV prefix on the verb stem, it either incorporates into the stem onset, deletes, or is incorporated into the coda of the preceding syllable, the latter incorporation places it in the penult syllable. In the traditional view of the template, the classifier is part of the conjunct domain (in pos IX) (see Chapter 2.6). For the study reported on in this chapter, it's affiliation is not important. The entity we are measuring in this chapter is the final syllable in the verb. I will refer to this as the Stem, meaning only the final syllable in the word. The Stem and the Verb domain are the same surface entity, their differences are in the structures they assume.

[2] The calculations are of the domains, not syllables. There are only 32 conjunct and 32 stem domains and 21 disjunct in the dataset. Each syllable was marked in the spreadsheet for the word that it was in and the domain it was in. The average is the average of the 32 conjunct and stem domains in the dataset, not the syllables. So let's say word x had a conjunct domain of 330 ms and a stem domain of 310 ms. But the conjunct was made up of three syllables and the stem had one. The stem syllable is 310 ms and its longer than the

conjunct syllables by a factor of near 3, the conjunct syllables averaged 110 ms. The domain averages are thus different from the averages of the syllables. (Note also that there could be considerable variation in the length of the 3 syllables in the conjunct.)

The conjunct made 54 contributions to its domain average (there were 54 conjunct syllables), versus 32 for the stem and 21 for the disjunct. If all the syllables were all the same average size, then the conjunct domain would be by far the largest domain since it had the most syllables. It's not the case. The syllable score reflects the difference the syllables in the three domains are making to their domain average. The question is, what is the source of these differences?

[3] Thus a case can be made that languages develop more complex gestures exactly because of the nature of their distribution constraints (McDonough 2002).

[4] See Chapter 1 for a discussion of the word lists and methodology used in the study.

[5] Speakers, wearing a head-mounted microphone, listened to a pre-recorded word list, and were asked to repeat the word after they heard it. Speakers were recorded individually, and there was variability in the speech rate and style since this was governed only by the recorded material and not by other speakers. It is for this reason that the original recitation of the word list used in the recording was included in the measurements of the data.

[6] In an earlier small field study of monolingual speakers, who were all in their 70's and 80's (headed by Martha Austin-Garrison of Dine College, Shiprock, N. M.), we noticed that sequences of nasal + vowel in the conjunct domain were notably compressed to long syllabic nasals, though we had not set out purposely to examine this phenomena. It is clear from listening to more causal speech that there are differences in casual and careful speech in, at least, the articulation of consonants and vowels. How these differences in speech style are determined by the prosody and/or morphological structure remains to be studied. However it is clear that the timing patterns we are seeing in the careful speech are particular to Navajo and will likely underlie analyses of more casual speech.

[7] This metathesis provides some evidence for an epenthetic analysis of the conjunct prefix vowels, outside stems from the mode or Base Paradigms (YM:g200). The prefixes are non-syllabic consonants, here *j*-. In this view, epenthesis accounts for the default vowel *i*- in these prefixes to the Infl stem, phonology accounts for the vowel quality differences among these prefixes (McDonough 1990, 1996).

[8] This figure was calculated over the 15,000 entries in the Young and Morgan dictionary that listed a Ib disjunct morpheme in its gloss. It does not count the forms in paradigms. See Sussman and McDonough (2002).

[9] There was a single word in the dataset that had an long vowel derived over the disjunct / conjunct boundary, *ch'ooshdeeł*, the optative form of 'I toss it out' (YM:d292). The gloss follows:

> *ch'ooshdeeł,*
> ch'í   # [ósh   ] [ł   deeł   ]
> 'out' # [opt/1s   ] ['cl' 'handle flexible object':perf]
> Ib   [VII/VIII] [IX X   ]
> D   # [Aux   ] [Verb   ]
>   *'I toss it out (optative)' (YM:d292)*

Chapter 5

SPECTRAL ANALYSES

5.0   INTRODUCTION

In this chapter I will be concerned mainly with acoustic analyses of Navajo vowels and fricatives. I confine the discussion to these two sets of sounds; they constitute distinctive aspects of the sound inventory and its integration into the system as a whole. The basic points of spectrographic analysis will be discussed as they pertain to the goal of providing a baseline description of these sounds as they are realized within the system.

In a generally assumed model, the acoustic production of speech is the output of two independent parameters: vocal fold vibration, which is the principle noise source in speech, and a filter, which is the configuration of the vocal tract above the larynx. For the vowel sounds, the vocal fold vibration is the source of the speech noise, and the configuration of the vocal tract determines the properties of the vowel quality. As seen in wideband spectrograms, the configuration is expressed by the lowest three or four energy bands, or formants, and, in a language, vowel quality and distribution can be determined by measuring the relative frequencies of these formants in the vowel phonemes. Fricative production, on the other hand, involves making a tight constriction–not closure–in the vocal tract. The area of constriction is narrower than that of a vowel or an approximant, and the articulation of a fricative can vary widely from language to language (Stevens at al. 1992, Shadle 1991, Ladefoged and Maddieson 1996). The fricative sounds, as opposed to vowels, are characterized by broad, random noise which exhibits characteristics according to the location and type of constriction used in the production of the fricative. In addition, for the strident or noisy fricatives, classically [s] and [ʃ], for instance, the vocal tract constriction causes audible turbulence. In voiceless strident fricatives, this turbulence is the principle noise source. The turbulence appears as energy in the spectrum, and this energy can be used to characterize the fricative sounds (Catford 1977, Shadle 1985, 1991, Stevens 1998, Stevens et. al. 1992, Fujimura and Erickson 1997).

In this chapter we will examine the acoustic properties of the fricative and vowels sounds using a spectrographic analysis. The first section of this chapter is an acoustic description of the formant structure of the Navajo vowels in the morphological domains. The second section of this chapter reports on the investigation of the spectral properties of fricatives.

5.1   NAVAJO VOWELS

Navajo has an asymmetric vowel space, and its vowel quality distinctions are extended by several prosodic features. There are four vowel qualities in Navajo, high and mid front *i / e*, round *o* and low *a*; there is no high back vowel in Navajo. The vowels exhibit length, nasality and tone (high/low) distinctions in the stems, though most of these distinctions are neutralized outside the stems in the usual Athabaskan pattern. In this section we will be primarily concerned with the spectrographic description of the Navajo vowel qualities, their length distinctions and distributional variation patterns.

5.1.1   The NavajoVowel Space

There is some variation in the description of the acoustic and phonetic properties of the vowels of Navajo. In Hoijer's (1945) study of Navajo phonology, he reports a phonemic four vowel system with both length and nasality contrasts. These four vowels are listed below in (1). Note the gap in the system; there is no high back vowel.

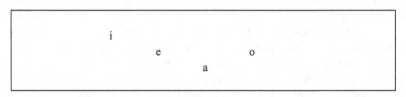

Figure 23 The four Navajo vowel qualities.

With contrasts in length and nasality, these four vowels provide sixteen phonemic contrasts, excluding tonal contrasts. The set of these 16 contrasts are listed in Figure 23: long and short for both oral and nasal vowels. The orthography deviates from the standard IPA symbols, as I have maintained the Athabaskan diacritics for nasality and length. Nasal vowels are marked with a hook beneath the vowel, length by doubling the vowel, as in Figure 24.

There has been discussion in the literature on the vowel quality differences between the long and short vowels. Many researchers have noticed that the long / short distinction has been amplified by a tense / lax or peripheral / interior distinction, though there is considerable variation in the description of the acoustic and phonetic properties of the vowels of Navajo.

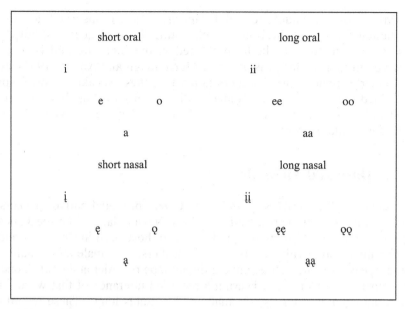

Figure 24 Navajo vowel contrasts (excluding tone).

Hoijer (1945:26-28) reports a quality difference between the long and short version of the high front vowel *i*, similar to the one in English. He also notes that the long and short versions of the mid front vowel *e* are similar to the lax [ɛ] in English, but with a higher tongue position before a high vowel. He reports the round vowel *o* is 'variable in quality' and may be 'pronounced as though the vowel were the cardinal vowel u' (Hoijer 1945:26); that is, he claims that the variation in the round vowel *o* that extends into the high back area, the 'missing vowel' area. He also reports considerable variation (fronting) along the backness axis of the low vowel *a*.

The Hoijer (1945) study is based on Sapir's data from 1927-1939 and his own 1941 fieldwork in the Chaco Canyon area of the reservation. The 1967 Sapir-Hoijer study, based on Sapir's field notes, reports similar allophonic variation in vowels, again noting a quality difference for the long and short versions of the high front vowel. In addition, this study notes that the *e* is a 'lower mid-front position'. Young and Morgan (1987) concurs with the Sapir-Hoijer (1967) study and, as in the earlier Hoijer study, reports the extension of the *o* into the high back area, 'especially when it is followed by *i*' (1987:xii).

Other studies of the Navajo vowels have reported different vowel effects. Young and Morgan (1972) report a quality distinction for the mid front vowels. Maddieson (1984) notes a quality difference in the long and short versions of both the *i* and *o* vowels and records the mid front vowel as in Young and Morgan (1987), in a lower mid position, suggesting that there are 6 vowel qualities, with a tense / lax distinction for both the high front and the mid back vowels.

McDonough, Ladefoged and George (1993) observed a quality distinction for all but the back vowel, noting 7 vowel qualities, but noted that this distinction was both unreported in the literature and is was not observed in their male speakers. The McDonough and Austin (1995) study of 4 elderly monolingual speakers noted that these speakers' vowel space resembled the vowel space of older studies, with vowel quality differences for the high front vowel only. They also noted that the mid and high front vowels were quite close.

5.1.2 Data and Methods

As noted, the speakers in this dataset were bilingual native speakers of Navajo, who live on the reservation and use Navajo daily. The speakers and the datasets used in this study are identical to those used in Chapter 4 and in the fricative study, with a dataset of 14 speakers: 10 female and 4 male. As noted, speakers were recorded into a digital tape recorder at 44.1kHz, one on one, repeating a word after hearing a recorded utterance of that word. The recording sessions were approximately 15 minutes long. These recordings were cut to a CD at the Eastman School of Music at the University of Rochester and transformed into .aiff files using SoundEdit 16. Because of the nature of the recording set-up, we did not go over the word lists with every speaker. Thus, not all speakers were comfortable reciting all the items in the wordlists, as noted, and the recordings were edited, deleting utterances where the speaker either did not repeat the prompt accurately or showed uncertainty or hesitation indicating a lack of comfort with the prompt, though minor speaker errors, such as a substitution of *n* for *d* in the conjunct domain, were accepted.

The speech signal was segmented and marked for its phonemic (rather than phonetic) values, with the exception of some of the prefix vowels as discussed in Section 5.1.6. As noted, consonants and vowels in Navajo have rather clearly delineated onsets and offsets, making duration measurements straightforward. The final vowel of vowel-final words tended to be closed with either aspiration or a shut down of the glottis, resulting in a clearly delineated vowel. Frequency values for the first three formants, F1, F2 and F3, and a duration measurement were taken for each vowel (chapter 4). Measurements for the vowel formants were taken at the midpoint of the vowel from a Formant Object in Praat, which represents a sound's spectral structure as a function of time, as a formant contour. To obtain this formant contour, the wave form was sampled by the Praat algorithm into 25 ms frames centered around time steps 10 ms apart. A frequency value for a formant was taken from the formant's center frequency, and formant values were taken 15 ms before and after the vowel midpoint. Females were sampled at a maximum frequency of 5500, males at 5000 Hz. Descriptive statistics were made on the midpoint values to determine the characteristics of the vowel space. As noted below, the vowels are divided into three sets: stem vowels, which contain tokens of the vowels of both noun and verb stems; conjunct vowels from the conjunct domain in verb; and prefix vowels in nouns, which exhibited auditory vowel co-articulation in some items. Three primary concerns of the descriptive study are the vowel qualities, the vowel specification of the default vowel *i*, and the influence of morphological domain on the vowels.

Because of the variations in the descriptions of the long and short vowel pairs, one of the aims of the study is to document the vowel quality differences between the pairs of vowels in this dataset of speakers. To this end, a non-parametric Wilcoxon Signed-Ranks test was used to test for differences along the formant parameters among the vowels in the data, using F1 as a measure of height and F2 as a measure of backness. Finally, it must be noted that the complexity of the language's morphology makes it difficult to find minimal pairs illustrating the vowels. All the vowels are in a CV(C) context, but other aspects of the context, including tone, are not strictly controlled. In the interest of providing a usable baseline description, I have presented the vowel data in charts demonstrating the positions of the three formants, and in data tables giving the median, standard deviation, range and IQR for all the vowel groups measured in the study.

5.1.3   Vowel Space in Stems

Since the stems are the only place the full set of the vowel phonemes occur, the stem vowels therefore represent the Navajo vowel phonemes. We will begin by laying out the descriptive statistics of the stem vowel contrasts, and their location in the Navajo vowel space. The Navajo four-vowel system, with its missing vowel in the high back area, differs from the reconstructed proto-Athabaskan vowel system, as well as many other Athabaskan languages, which are five vowel systems (Krauss and Leer 1976). One descriptive question concerns the symmetry of the vowel distribution: does this system maintain a gap in the high back area of the vowel space? Is there, in fact, a missing vowel, or does the system adjust for this gap, for instance, by making the mid back vowels higher than the mid front vowels, in effect skewing the system (Lindblom and Maddieson 1988)? The dispersion of the mid back vowel into the high back space has been observed by Hoijer (1945), Maddieson (1984) and YM (1987), who also note that this occurs when the back vowel precedes a high front vowel, though none of these observations were based on instrumental studies.

A second question concerns vowel quality differences between long and short vowels in this dataset. As noted, observations on vowel quality differences between long and short vowels differ in the reports on the Navajo vowel space. There is a consensus on the vowel quality difference between the long and short high front vowel, and this difference is easily discernable in the speech in this data. The distinction is clear enough that speakers will correct mispronunciation of the *i, ii* vowels, but not others. For the other three vowels, the mid front *e, ee*, the low *a, aa* and the back *o, oo*, there are differences in the reports of their qualities. The McDonough, Ladefoged and George (1993) study reported long-short quality differences in all but the low vowel for their female speakers, but not the male; in addition they reported distinctions in the vowel space of male versus female vowels sufficient to exclude the males from the study. That study was based on 7 speakers and a smaller dataset than the present one. A small study of 4 elderly monolingual speakers showed a vowel space more like that reported on by Sapir-Hoijer (1967) and YM (1987); there was a vowel quality difference between the high front vowels, and a mid vowel that was rather low, but there were no other vowel quality differences.

As stated, measurements of the first three formants were taken at the midpoint of the vowel. Table 31 provides, for the long and short vowel contrasts marked in the stems in the data, the median, standard deviation, range, and IQR (mid 50% range) for the formant frequencies in Hz and for the vowel durations in ms.

First note that there is an uneven distribution of vowels in the dataset. the short high front vowel *i* is the most common vowel (n=155) followed by the low vowels *aa* (n=144) *a* (n=111), and then by *ee* (n= 99), *o* (n=83), *ii* (n=54), *oo* (n=35) and *e* (n=29). Presently there is no way of knowing how accurately this distribution represents the distributional constraints in the lexicon, though the mid front vowel is slightly less common overall. I have chosen to report figures based on all the vowels in the dataset, despite the distribution inequities. For this reason I have given the figure for the median in the descriptive statistics. In Figure 25 is a plot of the median of first three formants for these vowels.

The figures in Table 31 are the figures for the vowels in the stems in the dataset, combining both noun and verb stems. Observe that the greatest difference between the 8 vowels are along the F2 or backness parameter. Note the difference between the front long and short pairs, *i, ii* and *e, ee* along this parameter. In a non-parametric Wilcoxon Signed-Ranks test[1] significant differences were found along the F1 or height parameter for the *i, ii* (p<.0001), *e, ee* (p<.0005), *a, aa* (p<.0002) and the *o, oo* pairs (p<.0276). Along the backness (F2) parameter, significant differences were also found among all the pairs. (In general, a lower F1 is a higher vowel, and a higher F2 is a more forward vowel.) In F3, there were no significant differences among the *i, ii, a, aa,* and *o, oo* pairs, but a significant difference in the Wilcoxon test was found in the *e, ee* pair (p<.0249)[2]. Thus the long and short versions of the four vowels differed significantly from each other in this dataset along both height (F1) and backness (F2) parameters.

As we can see from the chart, the long versions of the front vowels are more extreme (higher and more peripheral) than the short vowels in the pair, which are more central than their long counterparts. The short low vowel *a* is slightly higher and more forward than the long version *aa*. The vowels of the round pair differ more in their backness than their height. The greatest parameter of contrast among the eight vowels was along the second formant, as we can see in the chart. Thus, if significance is used a possible measure of perceptual distinctiveness, contrastiveness or vowel quality difference, then the vowel pairs in this set all show vowel quality differences between their long and short versions along two of their most characteristic parameters.

Table 31 The statistics for the count, duration (ms), and the first three formants (in Hz) of the stem vowels in the dataset

Stem vowels		*i*	*ii*	*e*	*ee*	*a*	*aa*	*o*	*oo*
Count		*155*	*54*	*29*	*99*	*111*	*144*	*83*	*35*
F1	Median	463	372	633	487	696	752	537	513
	Std Dev	118	91	101	89	161	129	108	91
	Range	573	520	417	423	771	605	569	500
	IQR	159	91	151	127	234	218	125	72
F2	Median	2057	2532	1882	2195	1454	1309	1154	957
	Std Dev	280	511	280	282	209	136	292	300
	Range	1909	2746	1504	1724	1150	1297	1244	1710
	IQR	390	428	206	406	293	145	387	98
F3	Median	2922	3129	2863	2894	2796	2744	2715	2781
	Std Dev	268	318	286	260	389	288	289	276
	Range	1479	1417	1204	1252	1911	1781	1430	1432
	IQR	289	467	319	319	507	328	397	288
Dur (ms)	Median	99	155	86	223	97	248	108	282
	Std Dev	36	74	24	63	45	75	43	53
	Range	247	286	112	317	324	420	201	274
	IQR	32	60	26	73	33	85	47	62

The values for significance across the vowels in the vowel pairs is also of interest as it addresses the second question, dispersion in the vowel space. Asymmetric vowel systems like Navajo's have gaps in the high back vowel area. Cross- linguistic studies of phonemic systems, such as the UPSID database study (Maddieson, 1984, Lindblom 1986) have established the primacy of [i, u, a] as the peripheral vowels. In a discussion of the UPSID database, Maddieson (1984) predicts that asymmetric systems may become 'skewed' to compensate for the missing vowel. In skewed vowel systems, the vowels shift, and the mid back vowels tend to move up and expand to

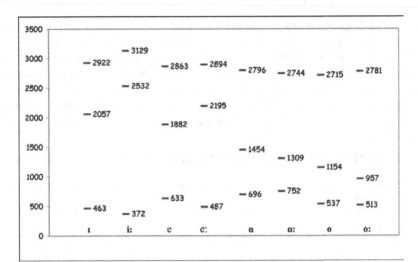

Figure 25 The vowel formants F1, F2 and F3 for the long and short stem vowel contrasts.

fill the gap, making the mid back vowel higher than its front counterpart. Thus if Navajo has a skewed space, we would find that the mid back vowels are higher than the mid front vowels.

In this dataset, no significant difference was found between the *e* and *o* along the F1 parameter; the front and back mid vowels were approximately the same height in the vowel space. There were, as expected, significant differences along the F2 (back) parameter (p.<0001). Furthermore, the vowels *e* and *i* showed no significant difference in backness, thought they were significantly different in their height (p<.0001)[3]. Of interest to the issue of dispersion in the vowel space is the fact that the front *i* and round *o* short vowels are not significantly different from each other in height (F1) (p<.0865), a statistic that it shares with the mid and high short front vowels. Thus in this dataset, the back round vowel extends into the same height space that mid front vowel inhabits, but both the mid vowels extend into the high vowel space. In the earlier study (McDonough and Austin-Garrison 1995), it was found that the front vowel space was very compacted, and the mid vowels were not mid-low as reported, but also rather close and high extending into the high vowel space. Thus a the Navajo vowel space does not lend evidence to skewing as it might affect the dispersion of the back vowels; however, both the mid back and front vowels in this dataset are rather high in the vowel space, and the vowel contrasts in the high front space in particular tend to overlap.

I have chosen to represent the distinction between the high front vowel pairs as *i* [ɪ] and *ii* [iː]. However, while we found distinctions between the all the vowel pairs, I've chosen not to represent the distinction between the long and short versions of the mid front and low and back vowels using different IPA symbols, principally because these differences are more subtle to the ear than the high front vowel difference, which is clearly audible, and which speakers are aware of and will correct. The symbols I might use to distinguish the long and short vowels of the *e, ee, a, aa* and *o, oo* pairs indicate quite different cardinal vowels. Instead I suggest that the short versions of these vowels are simply more centralized allophones of the long versions, while the contrast between the short and long high front vowel is more clearly phonemic. Thus these vowels are presented as *e* [ε], *ee* [ε:], *a* [ɑ], *aa* [ɑ:] and *o* [o], *oo* [o:], with the mid vowels high in the vowel space. In this study vowel context was defined across the word, and in an ANOVA test, there was no significant effect of word on the stem vowel qualities in the dataset, except for the high front short vowel *i* [I] (p<.0001).

Table 32 Mean formant frequencies (standard deviation) of the vowels of the female speakers of Navajo from the McDonough, et. al. (1993) study of 7 speakers.

	long	short	long	short	long	short	long	short
	i:	I	ε:	ε	o:	o	ɑ:	ɑ
F1	315	391	498	619	488	558	802	808
	(40)	(60)	(72)	(98)	(132)	(109)	(63)	(50)
F2	2528	2069	2200	2017	943	1176	1279	1299
	(279)	(256)	(124)	(149)	(143)	(243)	(122)	(99)
F3	3228	2926	2829	2880	2702	2843	2660	2314
	(279)	(207)	(213)	(131)	(477)	(374)	(392)	(534)
count	48	60	31	15	43	39	20	13

In a comparison of these formants values with those of the 1993 (in Table 32) study shows the formants values are similar for the front and round vowels, but not the F1 and F2 values for the low vowel pair, *a, aa* (a, F1= 696 vs. 808, F2= 1454 vs. 1299 ; aa, F1=752 vs. 802, F2=1309 vs. 1279Hz). The low vowels in the present dataset were slightly lower and more forward than those in the earlier data.

Finally, recall that assimilation processes in Navajo tend to be regressive, spreading features from the stem onto the preceding consonants and vowels. As we will see in Section 5.3.2, the stem vowels have a strong influence on the place features of the back fricatives, and the noun prefix vowel appears to be sensitive to regressive assimilation from the stem vowel.

5.1.4 Nasal Stem Vowels

The contrast between oral and nasal vowels occurs only in the stems. There are five nasal vowels in the dataset, *į, įį, ęę, ą, ǫ*. While no nasal airflow data was collected for these vowels, the figures for the first three formants of the nasal stem vowels in the data set are in Table 33. These figures were taken at the midpoint in the vowel. However, these values do not differ significantly from formants values taken 15 ms before and after this midpoint; the vowels in Navajo are relatively steady state in the usual conditions.

Table 33 The statistics for the count, duration (ms), and the first three formants (in Hz) of the nasal stem vowels in the dataset.

Stem vowels, Nasal		*į*	*įį*	*ęę*	*ą*	*ǫ*
	Count	11	85	25	21	11
F1	Median	488	375	562	705	539
	Std Dev	142	80	104	258	78
	Range	450	323	471	1236	220
	IQR	193	105	138	219	151
F2	Median	2331	2495	1948	1318	1075
	Std Dev	245	601	469	206	351
	Range	786	2683	1981	824	1093
	IQR	365	452	537	210	380
F2	Median	2983	3050	3026	2852	2929
	Std Dev	196	293	381	525	362
	Range	764	1195	1337	2044	1292
	IQR	175	436	369	749	460
Duration (ms)	Median	141	219	245	144	139

A comparison of these vowels and the oral vowels in Table 31 shows that these vowels have formant values that are very similar to the oral vowels. The main differences are in the F2 of the short high front and low vowel (*i* 2057Hz vs. *į* 2331Hz, and *a* 1454Hz vs. *ą* 1318Hz) and F1 of the long mid front vowels (*ee* 487Hz vs. *ęę* 562Hz).

5.1.5 The Vowels of the Conjunct Domain

The conjunct vowel distribution patterns are distinct from those of the stems; most of the vowel contrasts are neutralized, and even those that persist (some quality, length and tone distinctions) are favored values and the distribution of features is marked. The default vowel in the conjunct domain is the high front vowel *i* [ɪ], which is by far the most common vowel. Arguments can be made that, outside the Base Paradigms, the vowel quality is either default or predictable by context (Chapter 3). One descriptive question is the specification of the high front conjunct vowel. Is there a difference in the formant values of the short high front vowel by domain, given the distributional differences and default status of the vowel in the conjunct domain?

The figures for the median, standard deviation, range, IQR and the duration of the conjunct vowels in the dataset are given in Table 34. These figures were taken from vowels in the conjunct domains of the verbs in the dataset.

Table 34 The statistics for the count, duration (ms), and the first three formants (in Hz) of the conjunct vowels in the dataset.

Conjunct Vowels		i	ii	ee	a	o	oo
Count		*510*	*104*	*13*	*42*	*54*	*16*
F1	Median	414	354	558	712	518	500
	Std Dev	116	49	165	180	82	66
	Range	731	257	504	717	352	282
	IQR	151	64	293	302	111	61
F2		i	ii	ee	a	o	oo
	Median	2023	2540	2119	1674	1296	987
	Std Dev	309	354	209	304	237	142
	Range	2468	1900	635	1145	1104	638
	IQR	364	377	348	399	287	128
F3		i	ii	ee	a	o	oo
	Median	2949	2987	2870	2893	2749	2669
	Std Dev	289	276	196	274	292	273
	Range	1703	1204	620	1563	1685	1146
	IQR	298	467	298	308	392	247
Duration		i	ii	ee	a	o	oo
	Median	78	138	174	89	86	205
	Std Dev	32	45	37	30	28	46
	Range	235	255	126	140	121	174
	IQR	38	51	45	40	43	61

As with the stem vowels, the transcriptions used in the segmentation were phonemic and they were not sorted for context. The long vowels *ee*

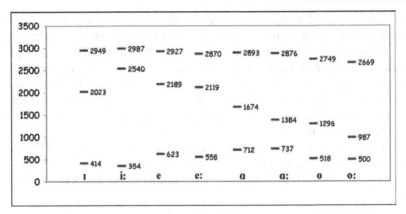

Figure 26 The vowel formants F1, F2, F3 for the conjunct vowels in the dataset (Note that the numbers for e and ɑː are not reported in Table 34 as they respresent a single token).

and *oo* were taken from tokens of a single word each.   Outside the conjugational forms of the Base Paradigms, all long vowels are derived. The tokens *a* and *o* were taken from a set of 5 words in the wordlists.

Of interest is the distribution of the vowels; the short high front vowel i [ɪ] is by far the most common vowel accounting for 68 % (510 / 743) of the conjunct vowels in the dataset, with nearly 5 times as many occurrences as the next most common vowel, the long vowel *ii* (n=104). Moreover, many of the vowels in the conjunct domain appear in CV syllables and have been argued to be epenthetic.   One question that arises with default and, particularly, epenthetic vowels is the nature of their specification.   It is possible, for instance, that these are vowels are determined by contextual factors, more than by their phonemic classification. This is a factor in a discussion of default values within the Athabaskan languages since the default vowel is not consistent across the family (see Rice 1986 on Slave, Story on 'Babine' 1984, Morice 1932, Hargus 1988 on Sekani, Krauss and Leer 1976, 1981, Leer 1982). If the vowel is variable or inconsistent, we would expect the variability to show up in the descriptive statistics of this vowel as compared to the stem vowels. We will see below that the conjunct vowels are quite consistent and furthermore have more in common with the stem vowels than with the noun prefix vowels, though the nature of this difference is open to discussion. We will take this up below in the section on prefix vowels.

The graph in Figure 26 is a plot of the median values for the three formants of the conjunct vowels given in Table 34.

If we compare the formant values of the conjunct vowels to the values for the stem vowels we see that they are quite similar. Using a Wilcoxon Signed-Ranks test, I compared the conjunct vowels to stem vowels of the same quality along the F1 and F2 parameters. There were no statistically significant differences for the *i, ee, a* and *oo* vowels on either parameter.

There were significant differences on both parameters for the *ii* conjunct versus stem vowels (F1, p<.0001, F2, p<.003). For the *oo* conjunct versus stem vowel comparison, there were significant differences on the F1 parameter at 5% but not 1% (p<.042).

Thus the default specification of the conjunct *i* vowel matches the specifications of the parameters of same vowel in the stem, and the default vowel specification as high and front in Navajo appears accurate. The variation between the vowels in the conjunct domain match the variation between vowels found in the stems, despite the differences in the distribution of the contrasts in the two domains and the timing and duration differences between the two domains.

5.1.6   The Default Vowel *I* and the Noun Prefixes

The noun prefix vowels are considered separately from the conjunct vowels for two reasons. Unlike the conjunct domain, which is an integrated part of the verb, the noun prefixes are more loosely attached to the noun stems as possessive prefixes. While nouns do not often appear without these, it is possible to ask speakers to produce a noun without the prefix, and the dataset contains several such pairs (*to, bito'*; *sǫ, bizǫ; his, bihis*), which speakers produced without hesitation. Speakers, especially naive speakers, do not have similar access to the verb stems. The second reason concerns the allophonic variation that can appear in the default *i* vowel in the noun prefixes. In the McDonough et. al. (1993) study, they excluded the prefixes in their data, which was primarily prefix-nouns, from consideration, because the prefixes were often extremely short, in some utterances not more than a couple of glottal pulses; there was more audible variation in these vowels. The authors observed that, given the variation in the default vowel specification across Athabaskan, and the shortness of the CV prefixes, the prefix consonants and vowels were likely to have different properties from those of the stems.

In this section we will consider the acoustic characteristics of the prefix vowels in the prefix noun pairs. In this dataset simple nouns consist of a prefix, usually *bi* [pɪ]'his/hers' and a (usually) monosyllabic stem. This was the form of around 80% of the prefix-noun words (see Appendix I). Recall that the noun word list from which these vowels are taken was constructed to illustrate the consonantal and vocalic contrasts as they occurred in the stems. The prefix was attached because it was common for nouns to have prefixes and because, with a CV prefix, we were able to examine the initial consonant of the stem in VCV context. Examples of these noun words are in (1).

(1)   bitaa'   3rd 'father'
      bijish   3rd 'stick'
      bit'iis   3rd 'cottonwood tree'

The vowels discussed in this section are the vowels of the prefix *bi-* [pɪ] in these constructions. With few exceptions, the vowel in the prefixes was the high front vowel *i*, and they were transcribed as such. There were two exceptions when the vowel was clearly and audibly not the *i* vowel; these vowels were found in the utterances *baghaa'* (3rd 'wool'), and *bowosh* (3rd 'cactus'), the spelling preferred by the primary consultants. These vowels were transcribed as *a* and *o* respectively and are represented as such in the data.

Table 35 The statistics for the count, duration (ms), and the first three formants (in Hz) of the prefix vowels in the prefix-noun pairs in the dataset

Prefix Vowels		*i*	*a*	*o*
	Count	135	14	10
F1	Median	415	584	443
	Std Dev	77	166	52
	Range	373	553	160
	IQR	107	215	82
F2	Median	2030	1287	1046
	Std Dev	338	174	284
	Range	1969	544	1047
	IQR	392	251	262
F3	Median	2901	2726	2762
	Std Dev	262	263	232
	Range	1437	1186	643
	IQR	280	230	448
Duration (ms)	Median	77	117	99
	Std Dev	27	41	37
	Range	127	131	121
	IQR	31	73	56

The figures for the first three formants and the duration of the prefix vowels of the noun prefixes are given in Table 35. There are three issues to consider: the acoustic characteristics of the default vowel *i*, the comparison of this vowel to the stem and conjunct vowel *i*, and the contextual variation in the vowels. As we can see in the table there are many more *i* vowels than there are *a* or *o* vowels, which each appeared in a single word. As with the

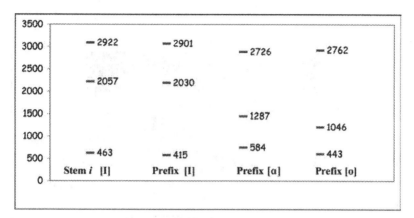

Figure 27 The formants F1, F2 and F3 for the prefix vowels versus the stem vowel vowel i [ɪ] (in the first column). The prefix vowels *a* and *o* are variations of the default prefix vowel *i* before stems beginning with a velar fricative + vowel, *gha* and *wo* respectively.

other vowels a measurement was taken from the midpoint of the vowel. As we can see from the duration figures in the table, the prefix vowels in this dataset, while they are short, are not extremely short. The median duration and the standard deviation is 77 (27) ms, compare this to the conjunct (78 (32)ms) and stem (99 (36) ms). While shorter than the stem, they are not different than the conjunct vowels in duration or standard deviation. In addition, in comparing the range and IQR of these vowels, prefix (127/31 ms) conjunct (235/38 ms) and stem *i* vowels (247/32 ms), the total range is considerably smaller for the prefix vowels, though the IQR is similar. If there was a great deal of variation, contextual or otherwise, in these prefix *i* vowels we would expect it to show up in the statistics for the range and IQR.

In Figure 27 is a chart of the first three formants of the three prefix vowels of this dataset and the formants of the stem vowel *i* for comparison (in the first column). The similarity between the stem *i* and prefix *i* is apparent in the graph. These vowels are not different from each other. As with the conjunct vowels there is more variation in the *a* and the *o* vowels across the three vowels sets (stem, conjunct and prefix) than with the high front vowel *i*. We can conclude that the front high vowel *i* [ɪ] is a stable vowel in Navajo, with clear phonological specification, despite being default by virtue of its distribution in the lexicon and status as epenthetic in the phonology.

5.1.7 Vowel Co-articulation

In a Wilcoxon Singed-Ranks test, there were significant differences between the stem versus prefix low *a* and round *o* vowels for the F2

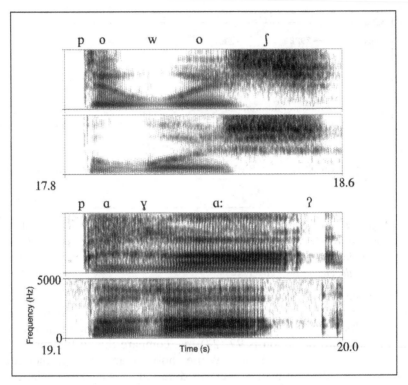

Figure 28 Spectrograms of the words *bowosh* [powoʃ] and *baghaa'* [pɑɣɑ:ʔ]: two female speakers.

parameter (p<.048, p<.009), though the value on the low *o* F2 was very close. The F2 values for the prefix vowels were lower than the stem vowels, indicating that they were more back than the stem vowels of the same quality. For a comparison between the conjunct and prefix low and round vowels, the vowels were significantly different on the F2 parameter (*a*, p<.0092; *o*, p<.046), and there were also significant differences on the F1 parameter for the round vowels (p.<016).

It is important to consider the differences in the vowel counts (stem versus prefix *o*, 83/10; *a*, 111/14) that contributed to these statistical differences. It may be the case that a larger number of prefix vowels may even out the differences between the datasets, but there is another distinction between the prefix and stem and conjunct vowels to consider; these prefix vowels were variants of the high front vowel *i* before similar vowels in the stem. Recall the words that these prefixes appear in *baghaa'* [pɑɣɑ:ʔ] and *bowosh* [powoʃ]. Example spectrograms of two speakers utterances of each word are given in Figure 28.

In both cases, the consonant between the two vowels was a velar fricative in its reflex before a back and round vowel respectively, as we will discuss in Section 5.3.2. The spectrograms in Figure 28 are examples of the prefix *bi-* as it appears before the velar fricative and a round *o* and back *a* vowel respectively. The vowels in the prefix and the vowels in the stem are identical. (Note also the final glottal stop in the lower pair; for both speakers it is a clear stop, with glottalization before and after its production.) Note the formants in the release of the stop, which are identical to the vowels formants. For the second speaker the prefix *bi-* [pǫ] in the top pair is quite short. Thus these examples are arguably cases of regressive vowel assimilation conditioned by the back fricatives. Note that there is little evidence of the effect of the consonant on the articulation of the vowel, as far as the formants structure shows, to the extent that the consonant articulation appears to be superimposed on the vowel articulation in these tokens. The verb dataset did not contain any instance of verbs with stem-initial velar fricatives followed by a low vowel. With the instances of a stem-initial velar stop, (such as *bił dzidíkaad* in Figure 29), the preceding vowel does not show similar coarticulation. This co-articulation reflects the variation we will see in the articulation of the velar fricatives in Section 5.3, and it is a quality of the interaction between the vowel and velar fricatives in Navajo that requires further study.

5.1.8   Summary of Vowel Data

In summary, there are five main phonemic vowel qualities in the Navajo vowel space, *ii, i, e, a, o*, as summarized in Table 32. The system has a gap in the high back vowel space, as the front and back mid vowels are not significantly different in height. The report that the mid front vowel in Navajo is a low mid vowel is not supported in this data; the mid vowels are mid high. For the stems, the vowel contrasts are extended by length, tone and nasality distinctions, making 16 contrasts, but these are confined to the stems. The formants values of nasal vowels are not distinct from the oral vowels, though airflow studies remain to be done to establish the degree of nasality in nasal vowels. The length contrast is often enhanced by a vowel quality difference, though this is only consistently reported for the high front vowel pair *ii/i* [iː/ɪ]. Outside the clearly audible distinction between the long and short high front vowel, I have chosen to consider vowel length quality differences as allophonic; the short vowels are more central versions of the long vowel pair. These findings are consistent with the data in the 1992 and 1994 vowel studies, thus the data in this section represents speech data on vowels from about 20 speakers.

Outside the stems, the default vowel *i* is by far the most common vowel, accounting for nearly 83% of the vowels in the pre-stem complex. This *i* vowel has stable values cross the domains, indicating that it carries consistent phonological specification as a high and front vowel. However, there is variability in its specification in the noun prefix *bi-*, with the stems that have back fricative onsets. This variability is best accounted for phonologically as regressive vowel harmony before the back fricatives.

Navajo vowels are generally more steady state than their English counterparts, with clearly defined onsets and offsets, even in final position. The vowels that show the greatest variability and formant movement are those that are surround the back fricatives, and we will return to this issue in the discussion of the back fricatives in Section 5.3.2.

There are several aspects of the Navajo vowels that remain to be investigated, including the degree of nasality and the contextual effects of nasal consonants, the effects of vowel quality on tone, and the distribution of tone and length contrasts among the stems.

5.2   THE FRICATIVE CONTRASTS

There are four phonemic fricatives in Navajo: three central fricatives, and one lateral. The three central fricatives are the two strident fricatives, the alveolar *s* [s] and post-alveolar *sh* [ʃ], and the back fricative [x], which is also quite noisy. The lateral fricative is *ł* [ɬ]. The fricatives are under several constraints in the lexicon. There are voiced and voiceless versions of each of the fricative sounds, though like English fricatives, the actual vocal fold vibrations is not a dependable aspect of this contrast (see also Holton 2002 on Tanacross). Furthermore, in Navajo the voicing distinction is not contrastive, but a contextual variation of the voiceless fricative in intervocalic position or after a voiced segment (Chapter 3.2.2). Strident fricatives are also under a regressive consonant harmony constraint (Chapter 3.3). Additionally, in some stems, the initial alveolar fricative *s* lenites to a glide intervocalically (Chapter 3.4). The back fricative [x] has range of orthographic symbols that are context dependent; this fricative has engendered considerable discussion in the literature as to its place of articulation and manner features, though there are no phonetic studies of it previous to the present one. These four sounds appear independently as fricatives but the same fricatives also appear as the release portion of affricates (*dz* [ts], *j* [tʃ] and *dl* [tɬ]), and as the release portion of aspirated plain stops (*t* [tx] and *k* [kx]). Thus, the Navajo stem onset contrasts can best be characterized by a distinction between simple versus complex onsets. Simple onsets consist of simple gestures (in the sense of Lindblom and Maddieson 1988) such as fricatives, nasals, glides and unaspirated stops; complex onsets are combinations of the simple gestures, such as affricates, aspirated and ejective stops, and onsets with the augmentative, all of which are combinations of stops followed by fricatives. This characterization is supported by the duration data (Chapter 4.2), which shows that the duration of the onsets is directly correlated with their complexity.

In this chapter I will provide a baseline description of these sounds using a Moments analysis of the fricative spectrum, as discussed below. I will also provide a measure of the voicing characteristics in a Points analysis. The first section will consider the three coronal fricatives, followed by a separate discussion of the back fricatives.

5.2.1   Methods

The same dataset was used for the fricative spectrum analyses as in chapter 4; this is a dataset of 14 speakers, 10 female and 4 male speakers, who were recorded one-on-one on a digital tape recorder, repeating a word list that illustrated phonemic contrasts and the distribution of contrasts in word structure, repeating isolated tokens after verbal prompts from a recording that was played to them. The collected data was then segmented and analyzed using Praat 4.0 sampled at 44.1 kHz (Nyquist at 22kHz). For the fricative study, two kinds of measurements were made. An LPC spectrum was made over the duration of the articulation of the fricative, and a Moments analysis was performed on the spectrum, using the parameters Center of Gravity, Standard Deviation and Skewness as a measure of differences. Visual examination of the spectrum was done using the LPC smoothing algorithm in Praat. In addition, a Points analysis was performed on the fricative sound as a measure of voicing.

5.2.2   Contrasts Between the Strident and Lateral Fricatives

Three phonologically distinct fricatives are under discussion in this section, the two strident fricatives *s* [s] and *sh* [ʃ] and the lateral fricative *ł* [ɬ]. This set of fricatives have voiced reflexes, *z* [z], *zh* [ʒ] and *l* [l] respectively. As noted in Chapter 3, the voicing distinction is weakly contrastive and is more properly considered allophonic than phonemic. Voiceless fricatives, which we may consider primary, appear in initial position in the word and after voiceless segments. Stem-initial voiced fricatives may appear intervocalically as well as after voiced segments. In final position and within the conjunct domain, phonologically both voiced and voiceless fricatives occur, though this is likely to be grammatical (aspect) marking (see the Base Paradigms, s-perfective conjugation, 1st- (*sé*) versus 3rd- (*iz*) person singular forms (YM:g201)). The context 'after voiced/voiceless segments' refers only to the stem-initial fricatives, since the boundary between the ultimate and penult (stem) syllable is the single place in the word where a cluster appears, providing an opportunity for a voiceless segment (*ł* [ɬ] or *sh / s* [ʃ / s]), as when the stem abuts a penult syllable with a coda.

There is little information at this time on the articulatory properties of the sounds of Navajo[4], and this study presents no new articulatory data. For information, I refer the reader to the discussion of the articulation of fricatives in general in Ladefoged (1993), and the cross-linguistic articulation patterns in Dart (1991, 1993) and Ladefoged and Maddieson (1996). These studies make several points relevant to the present discussion. First, I have classified these fricatives as acoustically strident; they are 'noisy' sounds. Articulatorily, strident fricatives are described as sounds whose principle noise source is the turbulence that occurs downstream of the fricative's constriction site when a jet of air, produced at the constriction site, hits an obstacle such as the teeth. This downstream turbulence is the source of the sound's 'noisiness' or stridency. All the fricatives discussed in this section (*s, sh, ł* and *x*) have this property; Navajo fricatives are generally noisier than English fricatives. Second, Ladefoged and Maddieson (1996:137) point out that these sounds require more articulatory precision than other sounds for two reasons: because small changes in the location of the constriction in the production of these sounds make an acoustic difference and, unlike stops or vowels, these sounds usually require maintenance of a precise tongue shape over the course of the production of the sound. Third, despite this needed precision, a great deal of variation in the tongue shape and tongue palate contact patterns in the production of the [s, ʃ] sounds has been reported in the literature (Dart 1991). However, the acoustic patterns in Navajo indicate that these coronal fricatives are quite stable.

For the purpose of this study I will consider the *s* [s] to be a [+anterior] fricative with contact in the alveolar region, and the *sh* [ʃ] a [-anterior] alveolo-palatal fricative with contact behind the alveolar ridge. The *sh* has contact that is wider and farther back than *s* and may involve more contact along the upper surface of the tongue, making it a laminal consonant. It also may be the case the *sh* involves considerable contact along the upper incisors, with a raised tongue body. Lip rounding, which is a property of the articulation of English sh, was not recorded for Navajo; however rounding is not a salient property of the articulation of Navajo *sh*. The lateral fricatives may involve broad tongue contact at the alveolar ridge, but airflow is along the sides of the tongue. Both the voiced and voiceless lateral fricatives are strikingly strident; the turbulence is a probable result of the air hitting the upper and lower teeth and the corners of the lips, and may involve the disturbance of saliva, resulting in spikes in the acoustic signal.

Figure 29 illustrates the main distinctions between the three strident fricatives in Navajo in two tokens of *bił dzidishkaad* [pɨł tsɪtɪʃkxaːt] from two female speakers.

First note that the three fricatives are quite noisy; all are marked by energy in the higher frequencies, showing up as dark areas in the spectrogram. The first major difference between them can be seen in the variation in the lower edge of the energy bands, which shows a clear

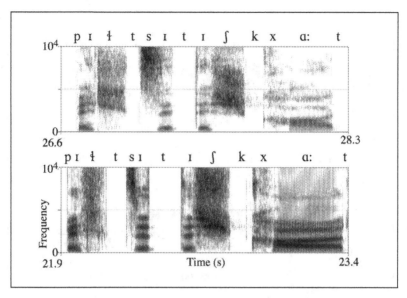

Figure 29 Examples of the distinctions between the three strident fricatives in Navajo: *s* [s], *sh* [ʃ] and *ł* [ɬ], two female speakers. Note consonant harmony does not affect the disjunct prefix *dzi*- [tsɪ-].

distinction between the alveolar *s* [s] in the affricate *dz* [ts] versus the *sh* [ʃ] and lateral ł [ɬ] fricatives. Note that the frequency range in these spectrograms is 10kHz. The *s* has a much higher energy concentration, with its lower edge centered above 5000 Hz in both speakers. Both the *sh* and *ł* have lower edges below 5000 Hz. The distinction between the lateral and alveolo-palatal fricatives is subtler, apparent in the amplitude of the fricative energy. In both speakers, the energy in the lateral fricative is weaker and more dispersed than in the alveolo-palatal *sh*, though their lower edges are approximately the same. Note also the distinctive spikes in the articulation of the lateral fricative in the bottom spectrogram caused by air turbulence on the saliva (Also note the velar fricative release of the *k* [kx] and the failure of consonant harmony to affect the disjunct prefix *dzi*- [tsɪ-]).

Because of consonant harmony constraints, within a word the contrast between *s* and *sh* is likely to be neutralized, at least when they occur within the core verb (Aux + Verb) or when they are adjacent to each other (see Chapter 3.3). One question that arises is the nature of the harmony process; is the *s/sh* alternation that is imposed by the harmony rule fully realized, or is it a partial process with, for instance, elements of an intermediate production? The spectrograms in Figure 30 demonstrate a harmony context. Note the differences in the location of the energy in the acoustic signal in the production of the *sh* versus *s* fricative sounds in two utterances, *yishcha* and *yisdzíís,* for one speaker. The *(y)ish*-, the 1ˢᵗ person form of the ø-imperfective, harmonizes to *(y)is*- when it is preceded by a [+anterior] stem, here *dzíís*. The frequency range in these spectrograms is 15kHz. The lower

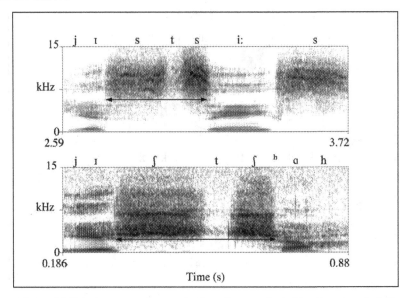

Figure 30 Spectrograms demonstrating the *s* and *sh* fricatives in *yisdzįis* (top) and *yishcha:* one speaker.

edge of the energy of the *sh* sound is around 3000 Hz, with another energy band at around 7000 Hz; the energy in the *sh* falls off at about 11 kHz. For the *s* sound, the lower edge of the energy band is quite high up, around 6000 – 7000 Hz. The midrange of the energy for *s* is around 10 kHz and there is still energy in the signal at 13 and 14 kHz. It is quite clear that these are identical sounds; that is, the regressive harmony is authentic. Also note that the release portions of the affricates *ch* [tʃ] and *dz* [ts] are identical to the preceding fricatives *sh* [ʃ] and *s* [s] respectively, and that the final *s* in *yisdzįis* is not visibly distinct from the other instances of the production of *s* in the word. Also note the lack of any voicing in the production of the central fricatives *sh* and *s* in these utterances.

The difference between the *sh* and *ł* can be seen in Figure 31, which demonstrates two examples of a waveform and spectrogram of a portion (*-dishłe*) of the utterance *k'idishłé*, for two female speakers. The sequence *-shł-* is marked by arrows in the spectrogram. Note the clear amplitude break in the waveforms between the two segments, marked by a line through the spectrogram. The lateral fricative has a smaller amplitude range in both cases and the break is clear in both the waveform and the spectrogram, though the lower edge of the energy bands are approximately equal in both the *sh* and the lateral fricative, as is visible in the spectrograms. Note also the difference between the two speakers. For the speaker in the bottom waveform and spectrogram pair, the lateral gesture is a voiceless fricative through only a small portion of its articulation, as marked; it clearly becomes a voiced lateral approximant. This pattern of a lateral fricative becoming a voiced lateral approximant was not uncommon in the data in

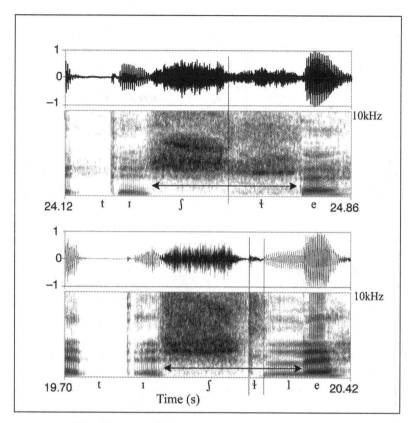

Figure 31 Waveforms and spectrograms of a portion (*-dishɬe*) of the utterance *k'idishɬé:* two female speakers.

stem-initial position, especially when the lateral fricative occurred in an intervocalic position.

These properties of the acoustic signal in the spectrograms discussed above are captured in the LPC spectra of these sounds. In Figure 32 the spectra for the three fricatives, *sh, s* and *ɬ* are presented. Each spectra represents 4 tokens of this sound from one speaker, though two different speakers are represented in the three spectra. The spectra display the distinctions we saw in the spectrograms above: the alveolar *s* has a peak at about 7 kHz, while the alveolo-palatal *sh* and the lateral fricative have peaks at about 3kHz. The alveolo-palatal and the lateral fricatives differ from each other in the amplitude of the peaks and in the broadness of the energy through the spectrum in the lateral fricative.

A Fast Fourier Transform (FFT) was performed over the duration of each of the fricative waveforms in the dataset to produce a spectrum, and a spectral moments analysis was performed on the spectrum. The Center of Gravity, Standard Deviation and Skewness were taken as a measure of the first three moments in the spectra.

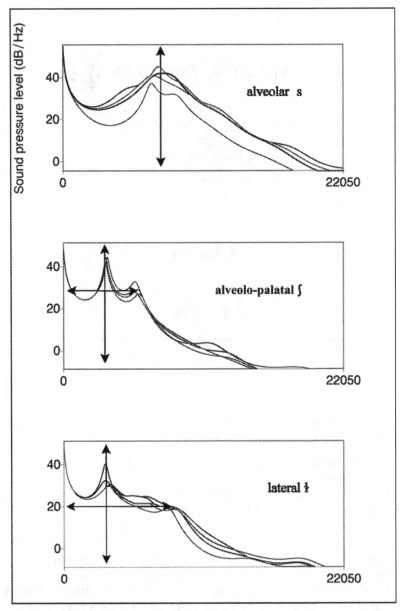

Figure 32 LPC spectra of the contrasts between the three fricative types, *s* [s], *sh* [ʃ] and *ł* [ɬ]. Four tokens each from two female speakers (same speaker within each graph).

Center of Gravity is a measure of how high the frequencies were on average in the spectrum, the Standard Deviation measures how much the frequencies deviate from the Center of Gravity and is used as a measure of how broadly the frequencies spread in the spectrum. Skewness is a measure of the shape of the spectrum. Statistics were done on these measurements of the fricative data.

For the alveolar fricative *s*, the Center of Gravity in the dataset was at 7kHz, the Standard Deviation, as a measure of the dispersion of energy, was 2752 Hz, and the Skewness was –1.04, indicating a high energy peak. The Standard Deviation of *s* indicates that the alveolar fricative had the broadest energy bands of these three fricatives. For the alveolo-palatal *sh*, [ʃ], the Center of Gravity was 3737 Hz, the Standard Deviation of 1423 Hz was the smallest Standard Deviation of the three fricatives, indicating a more compact energy, and the Skewness was positive at 1.42. The lateral fricative has a slightly lower Center of Gravity than the alveolo-palatal fricative, at 2413 Hz, and a higher Standard Deviation at 2136 Hz with a positive skew at 1.77. The lower Center of Gravity is an indication of the lower amplitudes of the lateral fricative versus the *sh* in general, the wider Standard Deviation indicates that the lateral had a broader energy band than the *sh*. These results fit with what we saw in the spectrograms in the preceding discussion.

Table 36 The statistics for a moments analysis of the three voiceless strident fricatives in Navajo.

	IPA	Center of Gravity	St. Dev.	Skewness	Count
s	s	6963 Hz	2752 Hz	-1.04	190
sh	ʃ	3737	1423	1.42	305
ł	ɬ	2413	2136	1.77	165

A posthoc analysis (Fischer's at 5%) was performed on the data; for both the Center of Gravity and the Standard Deviation measures, there were significant differences between all the three fricatives (p <.0001). For Skewness, there were significant differences between the alveolar fricative *s* and the *sh*, and between *s* and the lateral fricative (p <.0001), but not between the alveolo-palatal *sh* and the lateral fricative. This is as we might expect given our examination of the spectrograms and LPC spectrum above, if these are representative of the speakers in the dataset in general. The lateral and alveolo-palatal fricatives have similar skew, but the laterals seemed to have less amplitude and a broader energy spectrum. While I have not reported a measure of amplitude or intensity, there were significant differences in the intensity for all three fricatives (p <.0001). The lateral and *sh* also differed in Standard Deviation, again in keeping with what we see in the spectrograms. The statistics indicate that the Center of Gravity, Standard Deviation and intensity differences are all significant. Thus the parameters of contrast among the voiceless fricatives are as the spectra in Figure 32 demonstrate: the *s* has energy in the high frequencies versus the lower frequency energy in the lateral and alveolar fricatives. The lateral and

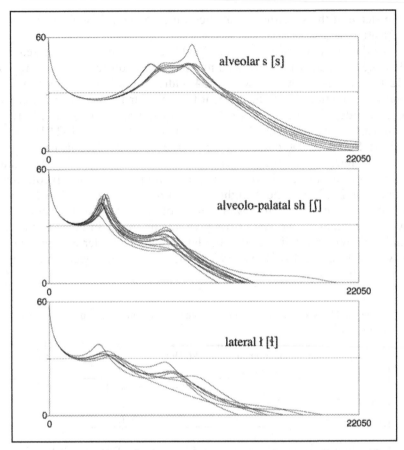

Figure 33 Superimposed LPC spectra for two speakers, alveolar *s* [s] (7 tokens), alveolo-palatal *sh* [ʃ] (13 tokens) and lateral *ł* [ɬ] (8 tokens).

alveolar fricatives differ in the broadness of their energy dispersion and in their center of gravity and their intensity. Finally, in the dataset of 14 speakers, the effect of speaker was not significant on the alveolo-palatal and lateral contrast nor the lateral and alveolar contrast, though there was a slight effect on the *sh* and *s* distinction (p <.0230).

The voiced fricatives tended to follow the same patterns, but these fricatives presented individual problems with respect to contextual voicing and I will take these up in Section 5.2.3 below.

There is one final aspect of the voiceless strident fricatives in Navajo that is worthy of comment. Throughout the literature on fricatives, phoneticians and speech researchers have reported variation in the production of fricatives within a language and within speakers as well as across languages. One striking aspect of the production of the strident fricatives in Navajo is their consistency both within and across speakers and across position in word, at least in this dataset and especially with respect to the two central fricatives. This consistency in production of the fricatives is demonstrated in the spectra in Figure 33. Each graph represents several spectra superimposed on each other of sounds *sh, s* and *ł* respectively as spoken by two female speakers and in a variety of contexts (from the penult coda, the stem onset and the stem final position). The top graph is the spectra for 13 tokens of the sound *sh,* the middle graph are spectra for 7 tokens of the sound *s,* and the bottom graph is the spectra of 6 tokens of the sound *ł.* Examples of the sounds were pulled at random from the sound files of two speakers and spectra were made of these sounds; the numbers of tokens reflects the distribution of the sounds in the dataset.

The spectra of the three sounds are remarkably consistent even across speakers and across contexts, including differing vowel contexts. The lateral fricative showed the greatest variation. As we will see below, the vowel context has a stronger influence on the back fricatives, and it may be the source of the variation in the spectra of the lateral as opposed to the central strident fricatives. Recall that the lateral fricative, like the back fricatives and unlike the two central fricatives, involves a tongue body gesture (Sproat and Fujimora 1992) and this gesture may be important in co-articulation with the vowel sounds. The consistency that these spectra exhibit demonstrate that the parameters of contrast discussed in this section are likely to be hold true in a larger study and may serve in modeling these fricative sounds.

5.2.3 Fricative Reflexes: the Voicing Contrast

The voicing contrast among the fricatives calls for discussion. It is well known that voicing in fricatives requires special adjustments in the vocal tract that may influence the acoustic properties of the sounds (Shadle 1991, Stevens et.al. 1992). Since descriptions of the phonology rely on the orthographic representations when there is no information on the phonetics of the sounds, understanding the nature of these differences is crucial to understanding both the orthography and the nature of the alternations fricatives appear to undergo. We will discuss some of these differences in this section. As noted in Chapter 3, voicing is largely contextual; these stem-initial fricatives are voiced in intervocalic position and after a voiced lateral fricative *l,* the only voiced consonant that appears adjacent to the stem. Voicing is contrastive in coda position, where it marks aspectual or conjugational differences, and the two lateral classifiers are distinguished by voicing, though the classifiers are under constraints that severely restrict their surfacing in a word and a classifier is often only present in the voicing of the stem-initial fricative (see discussion in Chapter 3.6.1).

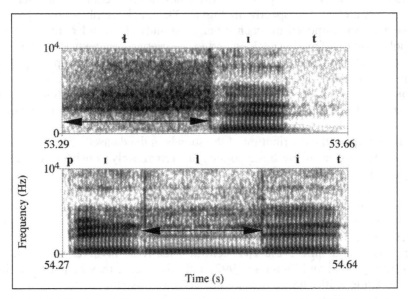

Figure 34 The lateral fricative in initial (voiceless) versus intervocalic (voiced) position: *łid / bilid* [ɬıt / pılıɪ]: female speaker.

The voicing distinction in the strident fricatives is demonstrated in the spectrograms in Figure 34, Figure 35, and Figure 36. These illustrate the lateral, alveolar and alveolo-palatal fricatives in Navajo by a female speaker in stem-initial versus intervocalic position in the utterances *łid/bilid* [ɬıt/pılıt] (Figure 34), *sęęs/bizęęs* [sẽ:s/pızẽːs] (Figure 35), and *shił/bizhi* [ʃıɬ/pıʒıh] (Figure 36). Note especially the voiced lateral in the bottom spectrogram of Figure 34, which is clearly an approximant with visible formant structure and continuous voicing throughout its articulation. The tendency for a lateral fricative to surface as an approximant in a voicing context has been noted in the literature (Maddieson and Emmory 1984, Ladefoged and Maddieson 1996). Note also the voicing bars in the intervocalic tokens of *z* [z] and *zh* [ʒ], the bottom spectrograms of Figure 35 and Figure 36 respectively. The stem-initial intervocalic position is the strongest voicing context. There is a weak voicing bar throughout the articulation of the zh [ʒ] (contrast the lateral fricative), and the voicing in the alveolar *z* is maintained only through the first part of its articulation.

Voicing in obstruents is different from voicing in sonorants because the constriction in the vocal tract has an aerodynamic effect on the vibration of the vocal folds; the pressure above and below the glottis becomes unequal, inhibiting voicing (Catford 1988). In voiceless fricatives, vocal fold vibration does not occur, and the pressure drop across the narrow constriction in the oral cavity is greater than at the glottis. The noise in voiceless fricatives has its source at the constriction site or, in strident

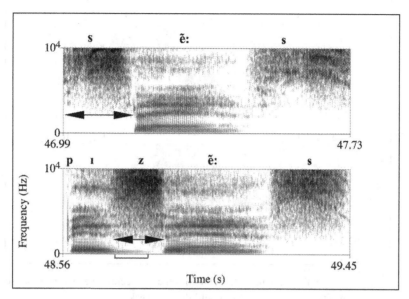

Figure 35 The alveolar fricative in initial (voiceless) versus intervocalic (voiced) position: *sęęs/bizęęs*[sẽːs/pɪzẽːs]: female speaker.

fricatives, downstream from it. In order to produce noise at the glottis, the vocal folds must vibrate. In order to get vocal fold vibration concurrent with constriction in the vocal tract the pressure above and below the glottis must be equalized enough to enable vocal fold vibration. To do this one of two things must happen: either there must be a decrease in amplitude of the sound source at the constriction site, or a change in the vocal tract shape between the glottis and the constriction site must occur (Shadle 1985, 1991, Stevens et. al. 1992, Stevens 1998). In addition, voiced fricatives may not be voiced consistently throughout the production of the fricative. Stevens noted a tendency of voiced fricatives to exhibit vocal fold vibrations at the boundaries of their articulation; that is at the beginning and end of the production of the voiced fricative, but the vocal vibration tended not persist through the duration of the fricative. Stevens et. al. (1992), Jongman et.al.(1994) and other have also noted that voiced fricatives tend to be shorter in duration than voiceless fricatives.

This model of fricative voicing makes the prediction that the spectra of voiced and voiceless fricatives may differ, since voicing involves distinctions in vocal tract configuration which are likely to affect spectra. To test for the properties of voiced versus voiceless strident fricatives spectral analysis of voice versus voiceless tokens was performed and several measures were examined.

The first measure of difference is duration. In keeping with general fricative patterns, there are duration differences between the voiced and

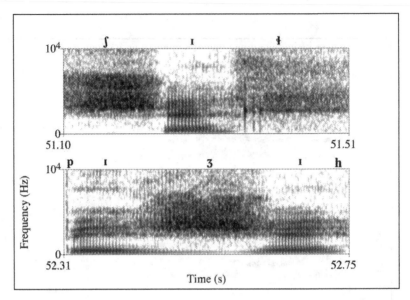

Figure 36 The alveolo-palatal fricative in initial (voiceless) versus intervocalic (voiced) position: *shił / bizhi* [ʃiɬ / pɪʒɪh]: female speaker.

voiceless strident fricatives in Navajo, the voiced fricatives being shorter. These duration figures are recorded in Table 37.

Table 37 The duration figures for the three pairs of strident fricatives in Navajo.

YM	IPA	Mean (ms)	St. Dev	Count
s	s	257.5	87.4	190
z	z	191	56	38
sh	ʃ	205	57.3	305
zh	ʒ	189.8	74.1	27
ł	ɬ	178.4	81.5	165
l	l	139.3	43.8	73

There were significant differences between voiced and voiceless fricatives in duration for the *ł* and *l* and the *s* and *z* (p <.0001) pairs, but not for *sh* and *zh* (p <0.2727). Note, however, that there are large distribution differences between these latter two sounds; there are 10 times as many instances of *sh* (305) in the dataset than *zh* (27), making comparison between them somewhat speculative.

A second measure of difference is a estimate of voicing. To get this distinction, an analysis of voicing was performed on the sound files of the fricatives using the Point Processing in Praat with a 10 ms window. The Points process counts the number of periodic intervals in a waveform as a measure of glottal fold vibration defined over the duration of a sound. Figure 37 shows the difference between the voiceless and voiced alveolar

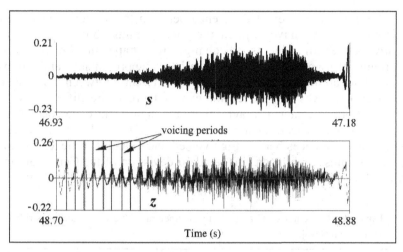

Figure 37 The waveforms and superimposed Points analysis of a voiced and voiceless alveolar fricative *s (point = 0), z* (points = 9) in the utterances *sęęs, bizęęs*: one female speaker. See text for discussion.

fricative *s, z* in the utterances *sęęs, bizęęs* for one female speaker in a Points analysis, which is superimposed on the waveform. The points were counted for the duration of the fricatives. The voiceless *s* is in word initial position in *sęęs*, the *s* sound is 252 ms long and there are no periodic intervals; the points analysis is 0. In the intervocalic fricative *z* (176 ms) in the utterance *bizęęs,* periodicity is present at the beginning of the articulation of the fricative, the points analysis counts 9 intervals.

Table 38 below gives the mean number of points for the three fricative pairs (the points are given without normalization for duration differences).

There were significant differences between all three voiced and voiceless pairs (p <.0001). The lateral was the most voiced of the voiced fricatives, and there were significant differences between the lateral *l* and the *z* (p <.0001*),* but not between the *l* and *zh* (p < 0.9380). The differences between the *sh* and the *s* (p <.0016) and the *sh* and the *ł* (p <.0034) were significant, but not between the *s* and the *ł* (p <.9371). The *sh* [ʃ] tended to have more voicing points than the two other voiceless strident fricatives.

Table 38 The figures from a points analysis of voicing of Navajo strident fricatives

YM	IPA	Mean (points)	St. Dev	Count
s	s	1.7	5.6	190
z	z	11.2	10.2	38
sh	ʃ	4.6	12.8	305
zh	ʒ	15.5	14.6	27
ł	ɬ	1.8	5.8	165
l	l	15.7	10.2	73

The third parameter of difference between the strident fricatives is in their spectra. We have seen in the spectrograms above that the lateral fricative especially seems to change its shape in the intervocalic environment; it appears to surface as a lateral approximant, and we expect this to show up in the spectra. Given the difference between the voiced and voiceless fricatives in general we expect there to be differences in the spectra. For the center of gravity there are significant differences between the three voiced fricatives as we expect (p <.0001), but there were also significant differences between the voiced and voiceless reflexes (p <.0001) of these sounds. The mean and standard deviation of the Center of Gravity for the three pairs of strident fricatives are reported in the table below.

Table 39 The Center of Gravity from the spectra of the three pairs of strident fricatives in Navajo.

YM	IPA	Mean (Hz)	St. Dev	Count
s	s	6963	1624	190
z	z	4159	2522	38
sh	ʃ	3737	546	305
zh	ʒ	2572	975	27
ł	ɬ	2413	939	165
l	l	894	1121	73

In the spectral moments analysis, the differences in Standard Deviation (2nd moment) between the three voiced fricatives z, zh and l, were significant (p <.0001). The differences between the voiced and voiceless reflexes of the lateral ł / l (p <.0001) and alveolar s / z (p <.0002) fricatives were also significant, but not between the sh and zh (p <.0387). For the measure Skewness, there were significant differences between the two lateral fricatives (a value of 1 versus 11, p <.0001), but not between the two other pairs s, z, and sh, zh.

In summary, there were significant differences in Center of Gravity for all fricatives. The alveolar s fricative had a high Center of Gravity, with a lower edge about 7kHz, and a broad energy band extending up into regions above 10kHz. The alveolo-palatal sh and lateral ł fricatives had lower edges around 3kHz, and they differed from each other primarily in the amplitude and broadness of their energy. For the lateral fricatives, there were significant differences between the voiced and voiceless sounds on all the parameters tested: duration, voicing, and the three spectral moments. For the central fricatives, there were significant differences in duration and voicing and Center of Gravity. For the s / z, there were also significant differences in Standard Deviation. The alveolar and alveolo-palatal fricatives were very stable in this dataset across speakers and contexts, and while the lateral fricatives were also relatively stable they tended to show more variation, possibly due to the fact that they also involve a tongue body gesture. In the next section we will consider the properties of the back fricatives, which exhibit a very different kind of pattern.

5.3 The Back Fricative

In this study, I have chosen to represent the back fricatives as the voiced and voiceless velar fricative phonemes /x/ and /ɣ/; this is a phonological representation. In fact, there is a great deal of variation in the production of these sounds by vowel context, by voicing environment, by speaker, and by morphological affiliation, in that order. My goal in this section is to present an overview of the general pattern of behavior of these sounds as a base for a further study, which will require a word list designed to illustrate these sounds under their different conditioning factors. Two principal observations that come out of the present study are: 1) the lack of a clear phonological distinction in manner of articulation between fricative and approximant and 2) a high degree of sensitivity to the following vowel. Both of these attributes may be found to be true of back fricatives in general, due to the physiological reasons: first, they share the tongue body as primary articulator with vowels, and second, their back cavity is relatively small, making these sounds likely to weaken or lenite in adaptation to context or to accommodation voicing.

There has been discussion about the nature of both the manner and place of articulation of back or velar fricatives throughout the history of the literature on Athabaskan. Hoijer (1945), while using the symbols for velar fricatives, consistently calls these back consonants 'palatals' and classifies them as glides: /x/ is a 'voiceless palatal glide' (Hoijer 1945:9), for example. Though he makes a distinction between /x/ and /y/ in place of articulation, classifying the /y/ as a front palatal, he also states that the /y/ is no different from the voiced version of the /x/ before /i/ (p15). In his study of Apache, the back consonants are also classified as palatals using the symbols for velars (Hoijer 1946:59), though he states that they vary (front or back palatal) according to whether they are preceded by a front or low vowel. Reichard classifies them as "postpalatals" (Reichard 1951:16). Sapir-Hoijer describes these as velars, which vary "very considerably in place of articulation depending on the vowel which follows." Sapir-Hoijer (1967:8). Kari (1976) and Hale and Honie (1975) refer to these segments as 'dorso-velars' and using the distinctive feature system of Chomsky-Halle (1968) classify them as [-anterior, -coronal], without specification for the feature [back][5].

The orthographic representation of these sounds in YM reflects this variation. The back sounds are variously transcribed using the velar symbols *g, k, k', kw, kw', gh* and *x*, as well as the symbols *h, hw, w,* and *y*. YM (xiii) classify these back consonants as palato-velars in their chart (xiii) but in the description they refer to them as velars. They write (YM 1987:xiv):

> gh – is a voiced velar spirant produced by raising the back portion of the tongue to a position so near the soft palate that when a stream of air is forced through the narrowed passage, accompanied by vibration of the vocal chords, a "growling sound" results, as in 'aghaa', wool, hooghan, hogan, gha'diit'ashii, lawyer.
>
> Before e/i. gh is so strongly palatalized that it is written y, and before o labialization is so pronounced that the phoneme is written w.

The orthography is a further source of confusion when the *w* and *y* symbols in YM are taken as labial and palatal glide phonemes, as opposed to phonological reflexes of a phonemic velar fricative. These symbols are used to represent both glides and fricative sounds in the orthography, though as YM state, phonemic glides are rare. The symbol *x*, which is the IPA symbol for a voiceless velar fricative [x], is used by YM only when the *h* symbol is preceded by an *s*, because, as they note, use of the *h* symbol here would cause confusion with the digraph *sh* [ʃ].

The velar alternation patterns are implicit in the orthography. In YM, the symbols *w* and *h* both appear before the round vowel, the *h* and *y* appear before the front vowels *e* and *i*. In both cases (front and round vowels), the *h* is used to represent the sound in its voiceless context, the symbols *y* and *w* are reserved for the voiced context in the stems[6]. In prefixes these sounds are all written as *h (hinish'na', hahodinishne')*. For the purpose of this study, I have chosen to represent these orthographic symbols variously written as *h, w, y, gh* and *x* in the Navajo orthography as the phonemes [x] and [ɣ] using the IPA symbols for the voiceless and voiced versions of velar fricatives, and allowing that the variation in the phonetic realization of these phonemes is contextual. In this view, sensitivity to vowel context and lenition to homorganic glides under voicing are allophonic properties of the velar fricative in stem-initial position in Navajo (and, by extension, Athabaskan in general). In this section I will lay out a general description of the back fricative patterns based on an acoustic analysis of these sounds drawn from the speech data in this study.

First note that this pattern of velar fricative behavior in Athabaskan reflects observations in the phonetic literature concerning the contextual variation of velar stop consonants (Sapir 1921, Keating 1988, 1990, Keating and Lahiri 1993, Recasens 1990). It has been noted that velar consonants tend to be articulated further forward before front vowels. This contextual variability of velars is arguably related to the fact that they share the tongue body or dorsum with the vowels as a principle articulator. Thus the tongue is pulled forward into the region of the hard palate by the front vowels, though there are differences across languages in these contact patterns among the velar and palatal consonants (Keating and Lahiri 1993). Furthermore, Keating (1990) hypothesized that for some velars this variability is not due to coarticulation but to underspecification. Velars are phonologically underspecified for F2, the backness parameter, and the surface tongue position of the velar is determined by the [back] value of the following vowel by a phonetic implementation algorithm. Keating (1988, 1990) and Keating and Lahiri (1993) determine that this underspecification is seen in the alignment of the main spectral peak of the velar fricatives to the F2 peak of the following vowel.

The descriptions of the velar consonants in the Athabaskan literature generally concur with these accounts of the velar stops. One question is how closely the Navajo data fits this general pattern of velar behavior.

The contextual variability of the back fricatives is a clearly audible property of their pronunciation, including the articulation of aspirated plain stops (see Section 5.3.3). I will lay out the general patterns of the variability of the back fricatives in this section, as a foundation for answering the questions that arise concerning their behavior. In particular I will attempt to provide a systematic analysis of their behavior as a basis for addressing these issues: do the spectral peaks of velar fricatives match those of the following vowels? Can the velar fricative variation be characterized as palatalization before front vowels, or are all fricatives equally likely to be shaped by the following vowel, indicating phonetic or phonological underspecification for tongue body position?

5.3.1   The Syllable-final *h*

Returning briefly to the orthography, one further kind of confusion arises with the orthographic symbol *h*, which YM use to represent two different sounds, as they clearly state: the voiceless velar spirant [x] "the voiceless counterpart of the gh" (xiv), and the voiceless glottal spirant [h], which only appears in stem syllable final position. The glottal fricative [h] appears as the coda of the stem of the word *kweeh* in the bottom spectrogram in Figure 38. Contrast this stem-final articulation with the final glottal stop in *biya'*. The glottal stop is a clear stop, with duration, complete closure and release. The final *h*, on the other hand, appears as a phonation type, as kind of post-aspiration on the vowel. The glottal nature of these two consonants is seen in the continuation of the formants of the vowel in the signal throughout their articulation (during the *h* [h]), and after the release (with the [ʔ]), indicating that the supra-laryngeal constriction of the vowel, its tongue shape, is not disturbed throughout the glottal articulation for either segment. The articulation of the *h* [h] is primarily indicated by the lack of voicing in the final portion of the vowel. In this way, the final *h* could be considered as a kind of vocalic voicing offset. The realizations of

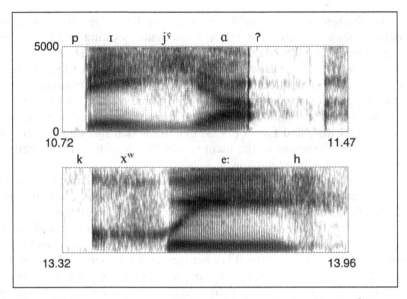

Figure 38 The contrast between the final glottal stop (top) in *biya'* [pɪjˤɑʔ] and the final glottal fricative in *kweeh* [kxʷeːh].

both the stem-final *h* [h] and the glottal stop [ʔ] demonstrated in these spectrograms are common patterns in the speaker's data. Thus the syllable-final glottal fricative *h* [h] is distinct from the other fricative consonants under discussion in this section, all of which involve supra-laryngeal constriction. (In addition, note that the stem- or syllable-final *s* [s], *sh* [ʃ] or *ł* [ɬ] are not distinct from their syllable-initial counterparts (Section 5.2.2)).

Notice also the formant structure and the fricative-like noise of the intervocalic glide in the utterance *biya'* [pɪjˤɑʔ] (because it is audibly more constricted than the English glides [j], I have represented it as a fricativized palatal glide [jˤ]), and the initial labialised velar stop *kw* [kxʷ] in the bottom spectrogram. The noise in the signal is consistent with some constriction in their articulation greater than that of a pure approximant. The glide *y* has the low F1 and high F2 of the preceding high front vowel, which is maintained throughout its articulation. There is clear movement in its formant values towards those which are characteristic of the low vowel *a* in the first part of that vowel's articulation. The labialised velar *kw* [kxʷ] has a F2 that approximates a round back vowel, and again this is steady throughout its articulation. The F2 rises during the initial part of the following vowel towards that of the mid front vowel *ee*. (The labialised phonemes *kw* and *hw* have distributions limited to front vowels; otherwise they appear as, or are neutralized to, their co-articulated counterparts.)

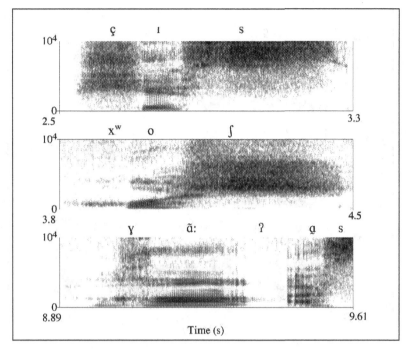

Figure 39 The velar fricative in word initial position in three contexts: *his* [çɪs] 'pus', *hosh* [xʷoʃ], and *ghą́ą́'as* [ɣɑ̃:ʔɑ̥s]from *ghą́ą́'ask'idii*, a female speaker.

5.3.2   The Acoustic Patterns of the Back Fricatives

The descriptions of the Navajo velars in the literature make two obvious predictions about the acoustic characteristics of the velar fricatives. First, they are sensitive to the quality of the following vowel, indicating that the formant peaks in their spectrum will be similar to those of the following vowel. Second, in Navajo, the stem-initial velar fricatives tend to lenite to approximants in the voicing context. Therefore we expect differences in the spectral properties of the fricative depending on vowel context and in voiced versus voiceless stem velar fricatives, reflecting their transition to approximants under voicing and possibly in their morphological affiliation.

The following spectrograms demonstrate the variation in the velar fricatives for one female speaker.

Figure 39 is an illustration of the spectrograms of the stem velar fricative in word-initial position from a female speaker in tokens for *his* [çɪs] 'pus', *hosh* [xʷoʃ], 'cactus' and the word part, *ghą́ą́'as* [ɣɑ̃:ʔɑ̥s-], from *ghą́ą́'ask'idii*.   Word-initial position is the position of phonological devoicing for fricatives.   The top spectrogram shows the stem-initial

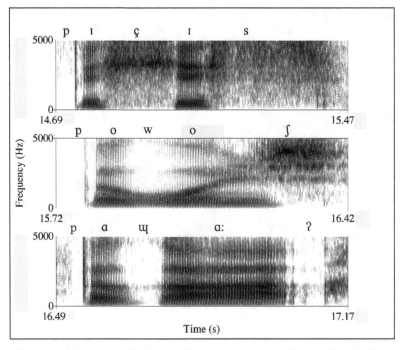

Figure 40 The stem-initial velar fricative in intervocalic position in three contexts: a female speaker (frequency range 5kHz).

fricative before the high front vowel. This is the most fricative-like of the three reflexes; it's lower edge of energy is around the third formant of the following vowel *i*. This pattern is characteristic of this fricative reflex in the data. The mid spectrogram illustrates the velar fricative before the round vowel *o*, which is rounded before the round vowel. The variation in the data is generally in both the degree of rounding and in the constriction; some speakers had labial glides for this segment. In this token there is a band of energy in the area of the second formant, though the segment is voiceless and is audibly fricated. Before the low vowel *a*, the fricative is partially voiced and shows the formant structure of the vowel. I have transcribed this as a voiced velar fricative [ɣ] in this context. For some speakers it is a clear velar approximant [ɰ], for others there is more frication in its production than we would generally expect of an approximant, at least of an English approximant. This reflex in particular consistently tends to have the qualities of both a fricative (constriction) and an approximant (formant structure).

In Figure 40 are spectrograms of the same three stem-initial velar fricatives in intervocalic position for the same female speaker for the tokens *bihis* [pɪçɪs], *bowosh* [powoʃ] and *baghaa'* [paɰɑːʔ]. The reflex [ç] before the front vowel *i* is nearly identical to the voiceless version in Figure 39: the sound is noisy and the noise extends high into the spectrum, the sound is voiceless and the lower edge of energy in the articulation of this fricative is slightly higher than that of the third formant of the following vowel. Among the three reflexes, the reflex before the high vowel behaves most like the coronal fricatives; it is the least voiced and most constricted of the three. In comparison to the alveolo-palatal fricative *sh* [ʃ], the edge of energy in this reflex is lower than that of the *sh* [ʃ]. This depiction is reflected in its Moments analysis.

Note the difference between this palatal reflex and the reflexes before the round and low vowels, in which the consonantal constriction is more approximant-like. I have transcribed these as the labial [w] and velar [ɰ] approximants. For the round version, the F2 format moves downward during the articulation of this sound, classic behavior for a labial glide (Stevens 1998). For the reflex before the low vowel, the F1 formant drops during the constriction. For both the round and the low reflex, F4 rises into the glide and falls out of it. Thus the primary distinction between the labial and velar approximants are in the movement and amplitude of F2. These two reflexes are, in effect, consonantal versions of the following vowels, and the lowered F2 is a result of the labial constriction. Both these reflexes are voiced, as opposed to the comparatively voiceless high reflex [ç]. One observation is that these two reflexes are lenited to approximants under the demands of voicing; the articulators are loosened to adapt to the aerodynamics requirements of vocal fold vibration. It is not clear, however, that this change is purely phonetic; it may be the case that glides are replacing the voiced velar fricative in the language. This is especially obvious with the labial glide in the data. If the blurring of the manner of articulation distinction between fricatives and approximants are characteristic of the back fricatives, then this is a property of the sound that is lost in some speakers, especially for the reflex before the round vowel.

Note also the harmony in the vowel in the 3rd singular possessive prefix *bi*; for these utterances the vowel has harmonized to the vowel of the stem, surfacing as [po] and [pɑ] before the round and low stem vowels respectively; an arguable instance of regressive harmony (Section 5.1.7).

The back fricatives do not appear in syllable-final position in Navajo, as do the coronal and lateral fricatives. These phonemes, which are the only non-coronals in the conjunct domain, are represented with the orthographic symbol *h*. Another question that arises is whether the sound *h* in the conjunct domain is similar to the back fricatives in the stems.

The spectrograms in Figure 41 demonstrate three reflexes of *h* (from the same speaker) before the three vowels in the conjunct. The tokens are of the conjunct prefixes *ho-* ('3rd area, space') and the seriative prefix *hi-*. The spectrograms illustrate the tokens [çɪnɪʃ-] from *hinishná'*, [nɑɣɑʃ-] from *nahash'ná* , and [-k'ɪɣ^wot̬-] from *bik'íhodiish'aah*. First, note that these are distinct from the syllable-final *h*, the glottal fricative in Figure 38. They all involve supra-glottal constriction, obvious in their formant structure and energy bands. Note that the pattern of variation is slightly different for the

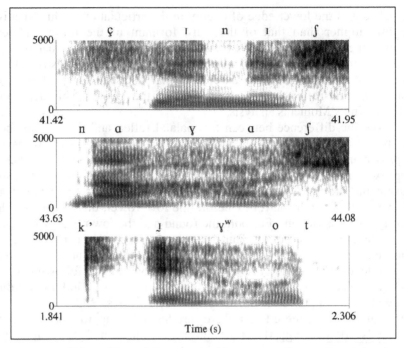

Figure 41 Spectrograms of the velar fricative in three contexts in the conjunct prefix domain: *hinishná'* [çɪnɪʃnaʔ], *nahash'ná* [naɣaʃʔnah], *bik'íhodiish'aah* [pɪk'ɪxʷoti:ʃʔa:h]: a female speaker.

conjunct vs. stem sounds. These sounds tend to have a more constricted, fricative-like quality than do the stem-initial reflexes, and this is an audible quality.

In the top spectrogram, for the palatal *hi-* [çɪ-], the low edge of the fricative energy is near the F2-F3 formants of the following vowel, and F2 falls as the vowel begins in a pattern that is nearly identical to the one in the stems. In word-initial position, this reflex is very clearly voiceless (there were no examples of a conjunct prefix *hi* in non-initial position in the data.). Before the round vowel (the bottom spectrogram) the drop in the F2 indicates the labial constriction, but compared to the stem-initial labial glide this articulation is more fricated, which is reflected in the lower amplitude of the formants of the consonant and the following vowel. I have transcribed it as a rounded velar fricative. For the low vowel reflex in the middle spectrogram, the formant structure of the fricative during its articulation is apparent, as F2 and F3 come together in a classic velar pattern. I have transcribed this as a simple velar fricative [ɣ]. The reduction in the amplitude of the formants during the articulation of these later two reflexes and following vowels indicate more constriction in the vocal tract than we saw in the stem-initial versions. Thus the conjunct examples of the velar fricatives are apparently more fricated versions of the stem-initial ones, less susceptible to lenition despite being intervocalic, but showing the similar patterns of context sensitivity.

We turn now to the statistical analysis of the fricatives in that data. As with the coronal and lateral fricatives, a Moments analysis was performed on these sounds. However keep in mind that the parameters of variation for the back fricative were greater than those of the other fricatives, and the word lists used in the study were not constructed to control for this.

Table 40 and Table 41 give the median, standard deviation, range and IQR of the measurements of the spectral Moments analysis (Center of Gravity, Standard Deviation and Skewness) and voicing (Points) of the back fricatives. The sounds in these tables have been grouped by the vowel that they precede. In stems, the voiced context is represented by the symbols *w* and *gh* as they are in the orthography, otherwise as the IPA symbol *x* is used for the phoneme.

Table 40 The statistics of a Moments analysis for the spectra of the reflexes of the velar fricative before the front vowels.

		Median	St.Dev.	Range	IQR
xi, n=30	Center	2779.0	1095.0	3992.6	1840.7
	StDev	2165.9	467.3	2575.9	511.0
	Skew	1.1	1.0	4.2	0.8
	Points	0.0	0.0	0.0	0.0
xįį, n=9	Center	3043.4	776.9	2428.6	1108.9
	StDev	1921.5	463.2	1439.4	663.8
	Skew	1.2	0.6	2.0	0.8
	Points	0.0	0.0	0.0	0.0
xį, n=6	Center	3429.0	1722.9	5137.4	1566.4
	StDev	2211.0	555.8	1579.6	319.3
	Skew	1.5	3.1	8.4	1.3
	Points	0.0	0.0	0.0	0.0
xee, n=31	Center	1915.3	1344.0	5590.7	2080.0
	St	1648.4	493.6	2108.7	659.3
	skew	2.3	2.2	9.5	2.7
	points	0.0	5.6	20.0	0.0

Table 40 represents the reflexes of the velar fricative in stem-initial position. For the reflexes before the high front vowels in the data, *i*, *į*, *įį* and *ee*, the Center of Gravity is around that of F3 of the following vowel (see Section 5.1.3), though the articulation is subject to individual variability.

For some tokens, the Center of Gravity falls to near that of the second formant of the vowel around 1700 Hz, but it is generally up around F2-F3 (2528-3228 Hz in the vowel data). It is slightly lower before the mid front vowel *ee*, as the F2-F3 of that vowel is slightly lower (2200-2829 Hz). I have transcribed this reflex as the palatal fricative [ç], in which the primary articulation is palatal; it is more fronted than a palatalized velar and more constricted than a palatal glide. This is also in keeping with the description in YM of the sound as very fronted. The measure Standard Deviation for the palatal fricative reflex indicates that the energy is dispersed throughout the spectrum. In a Points analysis, these show no voicing; again these reflexes before the front vowel pattern more with the coronal fricatives than they do with the low and round reflexes. The statistics reflect the tokens we saw in the spectrograms in Figure 39 and Figure 40; the reflex of the velar fricative phoneme /x/ before a front vowel is a voiceless palatal fricative [ç] in this data.

Table 41 The median, standard deviation, range and IQR of the measurements of the fricative Moments analysis (Center of Gravity, Standard Deviation and Skewness) and voicing (Points) for the back fricatives and approximants before round and low vowels.

		Median	St. Dev.	Range	IQR
xa/aa, n=46	Center	1368.3	551.5	1941.2	816.1
	StD	1102.6	459.1	2046.4	748.7
	Skew	4.3	3.5	14.1	5.0
	Points	0.0	5.2	19.0	5.0
gha/ą́ą́, n=18	Center	397.4	424.0	1784.2	200.2
stem	StDev	578.5	429.6	1496.2	374.8
	Skew	10.1	6.4	22.5	8.1
	Points	20.0	11.3	35.0	16.0
xo, n=64	Center	481.9	416.5	2133.2	349.0
	StDev	729.1	474.4	2581.5	417.1
	Skew	10.4	6.1	29.5	8.5
	Points	6.0	6.0	21.0	10.0
wo, n=16	Center	376.2	125.6	540.9	118.5
stem	StDev	305.4	321.5	1190.2	164.9
	Skew	22.3	7.7	27.8	7.9
	Points	18.5	10.8	44.0	7.0

The reflexes before the low and round vowels show more variation than the high front reflex, as their description and orthography indicate. In Table

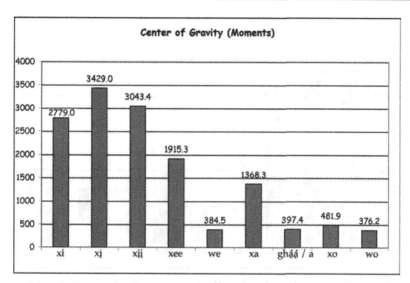

Figure 42 Chart of the Center of Gravity from the Moments analysis of the velar fricatives in the data, including a true labial glide from (*awee'* [ʔawe:ʔ] 'baby') for comparison.

41 the segments have been grouped according to their voicing environment. The tokens *xa/xaa* are devoiced, and they have a Center of Gravity that is around that of the second formant of the following vowel (1300Hz); the Standard Deviation as a measure of the energy dispersal in the spectrum is broader than in their voiced reflexes. The Points analysis indicate that these are voiceless velar fricatives.

Contrast this with the voiced versions of these reflexes indicated as *ghą́ą́/a-* in the table. These segments, written with *gh*, have a low Center of Gravity, a narrow Standard Deviation, and a high voicing index; these segments have formant structure; that is, they are more approximant than fricative. The reflexes before the round vowel are also separated into two groups, in this case stems (*wo*) and prefixes (*xo*). These two groups are very similar, but the labial glide [wo] from the stem has a higher voicing index and a narrower standard deviation than the prefixal reflex.

These results are presented in the charts for Center of Gravity (Figure 42) and Standard Deviation (indicating energy dispersion in the spectrum as a measure of frication; Figure 43) of the fricative Moments analysis of the data in the study. In these charts, the distinctions between the reflexes before the front vowels and the low and round vowels are apparent. The palatal reflexes are fricatives and resemble the patterns we saw with the coronal and lateral fricatives. These sounds are more constricted than the other reflexes and have acoustic properties of fricatives. The reflexes before the round and low vowels are more approximant-like, with formant values and the narrower energy more characteristic of sonorants. For contrast, the

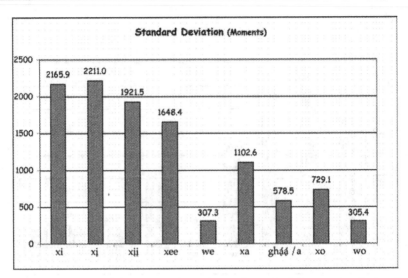

Figure 43 Chart of the Standard Deviation from the Moments analysis of the velar fricatives in the data, including a true labial glide from (*awee'* [ʔawe:ʔ] 'baby') for comparison.

values of an example of the 'true' labial glide from the token *awee'* [ʔawe:ʔ] 'baby' is given.

In conclusion, the back fricatives are phonemic velar fricatives with reflexes that vary in place and manner of articulation. This variation is tied to the vowel following the phoneme (front, round or low), the voicing context (+/- voice), and the morphological status of the segment (stem versus prefix). The general pattern is that the three reflexes all take their primary place specifications from the following vowels. The high or palatal reflexes are primarily realized as palatal fricatives and they tend to resist voicing in the manner of the coronal fricatives in Navajo. The reflexes before the low and round vowels are characterized by mixed manner properties; they are intermediate between fricatives and approximants and tend to move to more approximant-like qualities in the voicing context. The round and low reflexes tend to have more fricative-like qualities in the prefix domain, despite being intervocalic. In this view the Navajo phonemes of the back fricative sounds are /x/ and /ɣ/; they are realized phonetically as [ç] as the high reflex, [ɰ, ɣ, x] as the reflexes before the low vowel, and [w, ɣʷ, xʷ] as the reflexes before the round vowel. Finally, there tends to be some speaker variation, especially with respect to the production of the phoneme before the round vowel.

5.3.3   The Aspirated Plain Stops [tx] and [kx]

As discussed in Chapter 4, the aspirated plain stops *t* and *k*, in opposition to the unaspirated stops *d* and *g*, have the timing and duration properties of affricates. They consist of a closure period (coronal or velar) followed by a release period; the release period in both the velar and coronal plain stops is strongly co-articulated with the following vowel. The aspiration as a feature of contrast on these sounds is quite distinct from the aspiration which appears on the affricates, *ch* [tʃʰ] and *ts* [tsʰ] (see the spectrograms in Figure 45 and Figure 46). In addition, the release portion of the coronal and velar stops are strongly co-articulated with the following vowel, which is a striking aspect of the articulation of these sounds, particularly with the aspirated coronal stop *t*. We can see this in the spectrograms throughout the text. I have chosen to represent the releases on the stops as velar fricatives, that is, as an example of the velar fricative in the same way that the *ts* and *ch* have fricative releases that are not different from the sounds *s* and *sh*, as we discussed in the previous section. Thus, these sounds are represented as [tx] and [kx], and the co-articulation is a property of the articulation of the release as a velar fricative.

Figure 44 shows the LPC's of the release periods of an aspirated plain stop *t* as it appears before the high front vowels *i* and *e* , the round vowel *o* and the low vowel *a* (as it appears in the tokens *bitin, biteeł, bita, bitaa, bito, bitoo)* for two female speakers. These LPC spectra are not different from those we have seen with the velar fricatives, and they share with the other velar fricatives the property of being strong co-articulated with the following vowel. I have chosen to represent the reflexes of the *t* [tx] as [txɑ], [tçi] and [txʷo] respectively; that is, the aspirated coronal stop is a hetero-organic affricate (as Young and Morgan state)[7].

Since the principle perceptual cues to place of articulation are in the release burst of the stop and its effects on the formant structure at the beginning of the following vowel, and since the release of both stops is a velar fricative, a question arises as to where the cues for the place of articulation contrast might reside. Gordon (1996) suggests that in Hupa these may actually be debuccalized for some speakers, but in both the production and perception of these sounds, the coronal versus velar contrast in present[8]. Given that the duration of the release portion of these stops is quite long, these usual cues to place of articulation are likely to be masked in the aspirated stops by their co-articulating velar release, leaving the issue of how these sounds are discriminated open for further work.

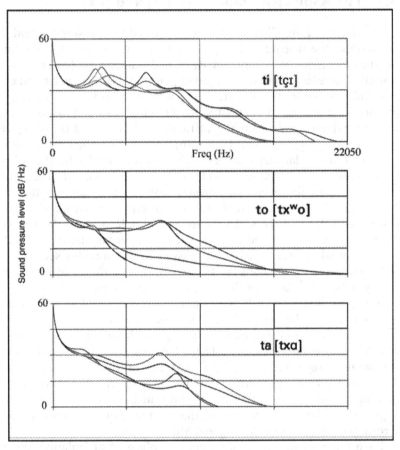

Figure 44 The LPC spectra of the fricative portions of the aspirated coronal stop *t* [tx] before the three vowels *i, o* and *a* two female speakers.

5.3.4 Aspiration in Affricatives

Another issue arises in considering aspiration as a feature of contrast in affricates. Affricates, as with all stops in Navajo, exhibit a three way contrast: aspirated, unaspirated and ejective.

There are clear differences between the ejective affricates and the others, as we have seen (section 4.2). This difference is illustrated in the spectrograms in Figure 45.

The affricates have a closure period followed by a fricated or lateral release, which like all frication, involves constriction in the oral tract. Note in Figure 45 that with the unaspirated affricate the vowel formants begin at or near the release of the consonant. With the aspirated affricates, there is a

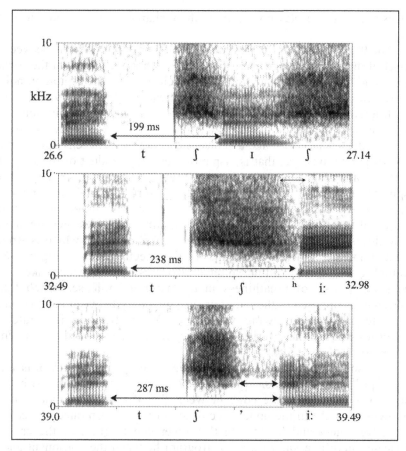

Figure 45 The three contrastive alveolo-palatal affricates (stem initial): unaspirated *j* [tʃ], aspirated *ch* [tʃʰ] and ejective (glottalized) *ch'* [tʃ'] in intervocalic position.

small period of breathiness between the release of the affricate and the following vowel. The ejective release is distinguished by its characteristic closure-release profile. The distinction between the unaspirated and aspirated affricates is the concern of this section.

   As noted in Chapter 4, the ejectives are marked by the particular quality of their releases, which has been observed in the literature (Lindau 1984, McDonough and Ladefoged 1993, Wright et. al. 2002). The release period for ejectives is similar to that of other affricates and distinct from that of the plain stops, by being around 50% of the duration of the consonant; that is to say, there is a considerable delay between the release of the oral and glottal gestures. With ejectives affricates, this means that the only air available to be used in the fricated release of the consonant is the air trapped above the glottis, and not, as with the regular affricates, the air in the lungs. We can see clearly in the spectrograms that this air runs out well before the glottal release, giving the Navajo ejectives their characteristic sound and timing profile.

For the aspirated affricates, there is a short time interval between the offset of the supra-laryngeal constriction, which is the source of the frication noise, and the onset of voicing in the vowel in which the aspiration noise is generated. This period is difficult to measure, but it is visible in the spectrograms. One way to think of this is to contrast aspiration in the affricates with aspiration in the plain stops. As mentioned above, Ladefoged and Maddieson (1996) make a relevant distinction between aspiration as a kind of phonation type, that is, aspiration as a by-product of the vocal fold activity, and aspiration as a supra-laryngeal gesture. I suggest that aspiration in Navajo affricates is of the first sort; it appears as a phonation type, a small breathy period at the end of the articulation of the release portion of the affricate. That is, it is essentially a laryngeal gesture and it is quite different from the aspiration gesture of plain stops, which is strongly fricated and has inherent duration. In the spectrograms in Figure 46 are examples of aspirated and unaspirated affricates by a female speaker. Note the small period of breathiness in the aspirated release, which I have indicated, as opposed to the rather precise boundary between the unaspirated affricate and the following vowel. This spectrogram illustrates the properties that are characteristic of the aspirated / unaspirated contrast in the dataset for all the speakers

The spectrograms in Figure 46 were taken from the words *bidziil* [pɪtsi:l] (774 ms) and *bitsii'* [pɪtsʰi:ʔ] (877 ms). Note the contrast between the two utterances at the edge between the affricate consonant and the following vowel. In the upper spectrogram of the unaspirated affricate, the two edges meet and blend. In the lower spectrogram of the aspirated affricate, there is a gap in the spectrogram between the consonant and the following vowel, which is most clear just above the 2nd-3rd formant (3-5kHz), though it extends above and below this gap as a small period of weaker frication or breathiness. In some instances, then, the aspiration in affricates clearly appears as a phonation type, a small breathy period at the end of the articulation of the release portion of the affricate. As noted in McDonough and Ladefoged (1992), this type of aspiration has proven difficult to measure in these aspirated segments, though it is obviously distinct from the type of aspiration found in the plain stops which, as we've seen, involves supra-laryngeal constriction.

Note also in Figure 46 that because the release period of the affricate is longer in the aspirated stop *ts* [tsʰ] than the unaspirated one, the aspirated consonant is longer than the unaspirated one (*dz* [ts], 234ms; *ts* [tsʰ], 341 ms). However, the following vowel is shorter in the aspirated consonant (300 ms) than in the unaspirated one (338 ms) indicating that perhaps this period of breathiness belongs to the vowel. It is not clear how consistent these consonant and vowel length differences and relationships are in the

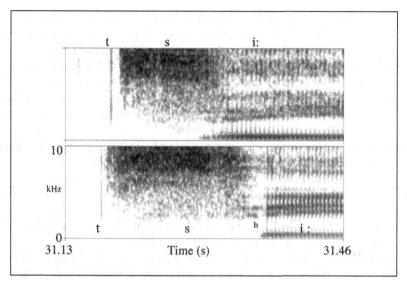

Figure 46 Spectrograms of the unaspirated and aspirated alveolar affricates dz [ts] and ts [tsʰ]: one female speaker.

data; this remains to be investigated in more detail, as does the measure of the aspiration in the affricates.

5.4   SUMMARY OF FRICATIVES

In summary, there are four phonologically distinct fricative phonemes in the inventory in Navajo: the two strident fricatives *s* [s] and *sh* [ʃ], the lateral fricative *ł* [ɬ] and the velar fricative *h* [x]. All the Navajo fricatives have a very constricted quality to them, as compared to English fricatives, which is evident in the ample energy bands in the fricative spectrograms. These fricative phonemes have voiced phonemic reflexes, *z* [z], *zh* [ʒ], *l* [l] and *gh/w/y* [ɣ] respectively.   For the coronal and lateral fricatives, the alternations are mainly voicing: voiced reflexes appear in stem initial position between two vowels and after the voiced lateral classifier (which is the only voiced consonant in this position).   These three voiceless fricatives can be distinguished from one other by the features of their respective spectrum. The voiceless alveolar *s*[s] has a much higher center of gravity than the voiceless alveolo-palatal *sh* [ʃ] and lateral *ł* [ɬ], with its center above 5000Hz, with a center of energy around 10kHz, and a broader energy band, with energy extending up to 13-15 kHz.   This is apparent in the spectrograms as demonstrated in the chapter. The alveolo-palatal *sh* [ʃ] and lateral *ł* [ɬ] have lower edges of energy in the spectrogram at about 3000Hz, and a more compact energy range, reflecting the fact that they are audibly distinct from the alveolar *s* and more like each other. They are distinguished from each other in their spectrums by their Standard Deviation as a measure of the broadness of their energy; the lateral fricative has a slightly lower Center of Gravity and a broader Standard Deviation than the alveolo-palatal *sh* [ʃ], reflecting its lower amplitude and wider energy band. This is arguably a result of its lateral articulation; that is, it has a tongue dorsum gesture as well as a coronal gesture and, in Navajo, the consonants involving the dorsum show a different pattern in production. In addition, as noted, the lateral articulation often involves enough turbulence to cause disturbance of the saliva. The central fricatives *s* and *sh* are only weakly voiced, at the edges of their articulation. The voiced lateral fricative, on the other hand, is likely to become an approximant in the voicing context, and in several tokens, the voiced lateral fricative shows a clear pattern of shifting to an approximant articulation during production; thus, the lateral fricative on whole demonstrates a larger voicing measure than the central coronal fricatives. Additionally, the central coronal fricatives are very stable in their production, exhibiting little variability across contexts or speakers. The lateral fricatives are also consistent, but they are less stable than the central fricatives and more prone to show variation dependent on context and speaker.

The velar, or back, fricatives have a different pattern. Their articulation involves the tongue dorsum, though their place of articulation is highly sensitive to context, hence the less specific 'back'. Like the other fricatives, they are considerably constricted during their production; they are, in fact, also noisy, though I reserve the term 'strident' for the coronal fricatives. Unlike the central coronal fricatives, they show considerably variability. For one, they are strongly co-articulated to the following vowel and thus subject to variation by vowel context. This is in part reflected in the orthography, which uses several symbols to represent these segments, usually associated to the vowel they precede, especially in their voiced reflex (= *wo, yi, gha*). These back fricative phonemes appear in one of three reflex patterns, determined by the following vowel: a high reflex, [ç], and low and round reflexes. The high reflex [ç] has properties similar to the central coronal fricatives, in that it tends to have a low voicing value when in a voiced context, and it is comparatively stable across speakers and contexts, maintaining a fricative-like sound. The low and round reflexes are more variable, with more speaker variation in their production; they have more approximant-like qualities and a tendency to lenite to approximants in the voicing context. This is especially the case with the round voiced reflex, which commonly appears as a labial glide [w]; this may in fact not be a phonetic reflex but may represent a phonological distinction. I have represented the round reflexes of the back fricative phonetically as [xʷ] and [w]. However, rounding is not an incidental property of the articulation. These reflexes are clearly rounded throughout their production, and this is visible in the spectrograms. The digraph *gh* is used for the velar fricative before the low vowel *a* in both the voicing and voiceless contexts when it is in stem-initial position, but as an *h* when it is in the conjunct domain. I have represented the low reflex of the back fricative phonetically as [ɣ] in both voiced and voiceless contexts, though it may also appear as a velar glide [ɰ] in stem initial position. For the low and round reflexes of the back fricatives, there is a distinction between their realization in the stem versus conjunct domain; in the latter these sounds are more constricted, and tend to retain more of their fricative qualities.

Apart from nasals, the contrast between a fricative and an approximant in Navajo is weak. In some speakers, the voiced back fricatives are quite approximant-like, likely due to the loosening of the articulator under the imperative of voicing. They show higher voicing values than the coronal and strident fricatives. In other speakers, a fricative constriction is an audible aspect of their production.

With respect to the manner and laryngeal contrasts, the distinction between the plain aspirated, unaspirated and ejective stops are best seen through their timing and duration profiles, as discussed in chapter 4. The release of the plain unaspirated stops are followed immediately by the onset of the vowel, but for the plain aspirated and ejective stop there is a period of closure, making them appear as complex segments. This means that the aspirated stop is not unlike the affricates; it has a release duration that is audibly fricated and co-articulated to the following vowel. I have chosen to represent this as a velar fricative, *t* [tx] and *k* [kx]; thus the reflexes of these segments are as follows: *ti*, [tç], *to* [txʷ], *ta* [tx]; *ki*, [kç], *ko* [kxʷ], *ka* [kx]. Thus, the aspiration on plain stops is a kind of a supra-laryngeal constriction rather than a laryngeal feature. With the aspiration on affricated stops, however, the aspiration is more likely a type of phonation, that is, it is a true laryngeal contrast, though this has proven difficult to measure. In addition, the velar fricative is used as a accompaniment to the stem onset as an 'intensifier', as in *łitsxo* [ɬɪtsxoh] 'orange'.

Finally, there are many questions left unanswered and much work left to be done, including a more precise description of the co-articulation facts of the velar fricatives, articulatory information about the tongue contact patterns in the strident and lateral fricatives, the type of phonation in the aspirated affricates, and the location and nature of the cues to place of articulation in the aspirated stops.

---

[1] I chose a non-parametric test of differences because of the highly asymmetric distribution of the vowels in the dataset.

[2] A Scheffe's (5%) posthoc test found the opposite, a significant difference between the *i, ii* (p < .007) pair and not between the *e, ee* pair (p <.96).

[3] A Scheffe's (5%) post hoc test, assuming normal population distribution, showed significant differences for F1 (height) between the two front vowels, but not the low (*a, aa*) or round (*o, oo*) vowel pairs. The Scheffe test also showed no significant differences between the interactions of the two mid vowel pairs (*ee, e, oo, o*) nor between *ee, i*. For

backness (F2), significant difference were reported for the front (*i, ii* and *e, ee*) and low (*a ,
aa*) vowel pairs, but not for the round vowel pair. There were no significant difference in F2
for the *ee, i* pair. Thus the Scheffe test predicts differences between the two front vowels, but
not the round vowels, and the low vowel pair differs in backness.

[4] Unpublished palatograms of some Navajo sounds are on archive in the UCLA
Phonetics lab.

[5] Discussion of the phonetic properties of these segments in the other Athabaskan
languages can be found in Goddard (1907), Golla (1970, 1977, 1985), and Gordon (1996) on
Hupa, Gordon et. al. (2001) on Apache, Holton (2001) on Tanancross, Wright et. al. (2002)
on Witsuwit'en, and Tuttle (1998) on Tanana. These studies indicate that the phenomena
under discussion is widespread in Athabaskan. The Keating and Lahiri (1993) study on
Russian report on a similar manner of articulation ambiguity in velar fricatives, indicating
that the lack of a phonological distinction between fricative and approximant in back
fricatives in Navajo is not unique.

[6] There is some variation in the orthographic symbol used to represent this sound among
Navajo educators. For the purpose of this book, I have used the symbols for the back
fricatives in the word lists that were given to me by the Navajo consultants on this study, and
they may differ slightly from those used in Young and Morgan. However, the transcriptions
in the examples taken from Young and Morgan are those given in Young and Morgan.

[7] Rice (1987), for instance, calls the aspiration of the plain coronal stops in Slavey,
velarization, and writes these as $[t^x]$. This is likely due to the same phenomena as we find in
Navajo, though no phonetic studies have been done. The prediction is that the aspirated
coronal stops in Slavey are likely to be as they are in Navajo, hetero-organic affricates, i.e.
coronal stops with a velar release, and the velar release is palatalized, labialised or
pharyngealized in the context of the appropriate vowel.

[8] I have transcribed the ejective plain stops *t'* and *k'* as [t'] and [k'], though theses
sounds have properties similar to the aspirated stops, the release portion is heavily aspirated
or fricated. This study did not report on the properties of these releases, though a cursory
investigation indicates that release of the plain stops is longer and more intense than a simple
release burst; constricted releases are a general pattern in the language. These plain ejectives
may well be represented as [tx'] and [kx'].

Chapter 6

HOW TO USE YOUNG AND MORGAN'S

THE NAVAJO LANGUAGE

6.0   INTRODUCTION

Young and Morgan's *The Navajo Language* is a comprehensive and multifaceted work of considerable significance to scholars and students of Navajo and Athabaskan alike, as well as researchers in the language sciences. We have only begun to understand and appreciate its value and scope beyond its important role in documenting the Navajo language. However, despite its being well-organized and intuitive, the volume is quite dense and not well laid out visually. Unless one is familiar with its structure and assumptions, its density can make it difficult to use. This chapter is intended as a tutorial on the 1987 version of *The Navajo Language*, and is best used with a copy of the 1987 edition in hand. I have included a tutorial chapter because of the significance of *The Navajo Language* to the study of Athabaskan in general and to this monograph in particular.

A full discussion of *The Navajo Language* is beyond the scope of a single chapter, and the work itself is only one of several grammars and lexicons that Young and Morgan have produced. The goal is to make the reader comfortable enough to explore the grammar[1], to understand the paradigms in it and how they work, and to use it to construct words.

6.1   THE YOUNG AND MORGAN GRAMMARS

The volumes of Young and Morgan's opus on the Navajo language (Young and Morgan 1943, 1946, 1951, 1976, 1980, 1987, Young and Morgan, and Midgette 1992, Young 2000) are the standard reference grammars on Navajo. These works make Navajo one of the best documented languages in the world, and by far the best documented among the indigenous languages of the western hemisphere. The opus is a complex and masterful work, akin in scope to the compilation of a major dictionary of English, such as the OED, but also containing a grammar. These works represent an extraordinary intellectual achievement, not only for their being a substantial grammar and a dependable dictionary, full of explicit examples of word use, but because Navajo is polysynthetic and morphologically productive. These types of languages present special difficulties in the construction of dictionaries, in part because our notions of what a dictionary is, and of what a mental lexicon is, derive from languages like English where words are simple entities, and word formation, while a productive component of the grammar, is limited in scope. We think of finite lists of words in English, and when word acquisition, word proccesing is discussed, the common reference is to nouns which by nature are generally less complex entities than verbs. English morphology does not have the extensive productivity or the ability to build propositions that are the outstanding characteristics of morphology in the Athabaskan languages. Athabaskan is a noun-poor language; the lexicon is primarily verbal. It is not clear what it means to talk of a dictionary in Athabaskan, or of word lists, nor is it clear what is stored in the lexicon, or how it is organized. In *The Navajo Language*, the dictionary is word-based, not stem-based or prefix-based, and paradigms are the key to word formation. The system is simple and elegant; there is a great deal to learn from the structure of the grammar. In no small way, YM's *The Navajo Language* is an articulated theory of the lexicon for a language with complex, highly productive morphology.

The main objective of this tutorial is to introduce the reader to the structure of the grammar by demonstrating how a fully inflected Navajo verb form is constructed using the grammar.

Because of the extensive sets of morphemes that make up a verb, Navajo and the Athabaskan languages in general are often characterized by a position class or 'slot-and-filler' template. This template serves the purpose of maintaining order among the verbal morphemes by means of a prosthesis of numbered positions. The positions are in effect place holders, and the template is useful for keeping track of Athabaskan's mainly prefixal verbal morphemes.

The extensive and productive prefixal morphology presents a number of immediate technical problems to dictionary building. If the dictionary is to list words in Navajo, then it must list inflected forms. Since a verb form is a proposition, the dictionary must contain a list of propositions. The main content part of a Navajo verb, the stem, may not occur without inflection, which always occurs to the left of the stem. Thus, a word-based alphabetic dictionary will necessarily list words organized by their inflectional prefixes. The number of distinct inflectional sound forms is small and the syllable shape is largely constrained to Ci-. Conceptually, this is akin to providing a dictionary of English sentences that all begin with pronouns. In fact, the differences between productivity at sentence level and productivity at word level in a grammar are significant to the design and structure of the grammar, and a study of the design and variation in the verb in Athabaskan languages demonstrate the nature of this difference. It is in this sense that the Athabaskan languages are important to our knowledge of grammar, because they represent a type of language that can inform and shape linguistic theory

The Navajo Language, 1980, 1987, *An Analytic Lexicon of Navajo* (with Sally Midgette) 1992, and *The Navajo Verb System: An Overview* (Young 2000), constitute the main part of the Young and Morgan opus. The 1987 *The Navajo Language* is a revision of the 1980 work, with some small technical changes, most obviously in the position class template (The 1987 template chart has fewer disjunct slots than the 1980 one, but they both have the same general structure and organization, as do all the template models of Athabaskan despite the differences in the number of positions they propose, and the 1980 and 1987 versions can safely be used interchangeably.). In this paper, I'll lay out the structure of the YM volumes, using the 1987 (YM) grammar as the primary grammar; unless noted otherwise, all references are to the 1987 volume.

The 1980 and 1987 grammars are both called *The Navajo Language*, and they are each divided into two distinct books within the volume, a grammar of Navajo and a dictionary. The grammar and the dictionary are numbered separately. In order to avoid confusion, I will refer to page numbers by the prefix 'g' for the grammar section and 'd' for dictionary section. The grammar section of YM 1987 runs 437 pages. The dictionary follows the grammar and comprises the bulk of the volume, numbered pages d1-1069. The dictionary is both Navajo-English and English-Navajo, though the former takes up most of the book. We'll begin with a discussion of the grammar. Since I will refer to the 1987 edition extensively throughout by page numbers and through examples taken from the book, this chapter is best read with a copy of the 1987 grammar in hand.

Figure 47 is an example of a discussion from the grammar section of YM87, in this case information about certain conditions under which the s-perfective deletes. Figure 48 and Figure 49 provide, respectively, an example dictionary entry and a prefix entry in the dictionary section of the grammar. We will discuss these entries in the following sections. Note that all three figures have been formatted to look as much like the original YM entries as possible, including preserving line-breaks, paragraph structure, and indentation.

6.2 THE GRAMMAR

The grammar comprises the first third of the book, pages numbered g1-437. In the introduction to *The Navajo Language*, Young and Morgan call this first section a 'grammatical sketch' that provides a 'wide range of detail' on the language. For every morpheme discussed in the grammar, and every word listed in the dictionary, several examples of its use are provided (see Figure 48 and Figure 49). The level of detail in this grammatical sketch makes this a significant source of information on all aspects of the language including its morphological structure. Because of the typeface and density of the text, when reading the grammar it is helpful to have a copy of the Table of Contents in hand (pages vi-xi), for page reference and to stay oriented in the text. If the volume were expanded to standard typeface and the examples listed in blocks, and organized with headers, rather than as it is as we see in Figure 47 and Figure 48, with the examples included in the text, the grammar would take up several volumes.

```
 Si-Perfective Deletes under certain conditions when
followed by ø-classifier and a y-initial stem:
   (a) If preceded by a di-VIa or ni-VIb prefix: deeyá
(not deezyá*), he has started to go, he's on his way;
neeyá (not neezyá*), he grew up.
   (b) If it is preceded by a low tone Disjunct prefix:
na¹-Ib = naayá (not naazá) he went, made a round trip;
ha-²Ib = yąąh haayá (not haazyá*), he climbed up it (as up
a ladder).
   (Cf. first person sgl déyá, I've started to go; néyá,
I grew up; niséyá, I made a round trip; bąąh hasáyá, I
climbed up it.)
```

Figure 47 A discussion of the s-perfective in the grammar section (YM:g153). The text has been formatted to appear as much like YM as possible.

```
      hahashshood (I), hanáhásho' (R), haháshóód (P), hahideesh-
      shoł (F), hahóshshood (O) (ł), to drag them up out one
      after another. Tsinaabąąs siziníjį' łįį' bee chizh
      hahashshoodgo hééł 'ííshłaa, dragging piece after piece
      of firewood up with a horse to where the wagon was
      standing I loaded it in./ (*ł-zhood = shood: to drag.)
      (hahi-.)
(391)
```

Figure 48 Dictionary entry, right column (YM:d393). Note center line.

```
hahi -²: ha - Pos. Ib, up, out + hi - / yi -, Pos. VIa-c. The
    hi - prefix behaves much like the seriative hi -, with a few
    exceptions, but it is apparently distinct.
```

Figure 49 Prefix entry, left column (YM:d392) referred to at the bottom of the entry in Figure 48.

The grammar section is divided into two parts, the main grammar and the appendixes, discussed separately below. The grammar section is preceded by three short sections: a bibliography (x-xi), phonemic inventory (xii-xv) and a preliminary section on nouns in Navajo (g1-36). The main grammar has two main subsections, on verbal morphology and on aspect. The verbal morphology is covered on pages g37-g139, and aspect from pages g140-g205. The appendixes provide paradigm charts, tables, and stem indexes. The term appendix is somewhat misleading, since the information in the appendixes play an important role in word formation.

6.2.1 The Verb

To begin, we'll briefly lay out the main parts of the verb. In (1) is a schematic diagram of the Navajo verb, which is comprised of three domains called the 'disjunct', the 'conjunct' and the verb stem.

(1)   [Disjunct # Conjunct / Verb Stem]Verb Word
          1   2   3

The internal structure of the domains is a controversial aspect of Athabaskan morphology and word formation. YM takes two approaches to the problem: they provide a position class template for reference, but they use paradigms to construct forms. The paradigms and position classes arre not isomorphic: they do not map onto each other one-to-one. The paradigms are compress groups of positions classes, reflecting the often polysynthetic nature of the paradigm form. They are provided because many template positions are abstract, in the sense that the morpheme combinations are not agglutinative or string-like, but polysynthetic. So in a real sense word formation in YM proceeds as follows: the position class morphemes are grouped into paradigms in a regular and consistent way, which they discuss and demonstrate throughout the grammar, and the forms from paradigms are combined into words. The goal of this chapter is to demonstrate how YM accomplishes this task.

However, the template is an important device. We will use the template on g37-8, as YM does, as a reference point. The positions are numbered by Roman numerals as in Young and Morgan, left to right, and can be seen in Table 42.

The positions VII-X are obligatory in the sense that they represent the minimal morphosyntactic specification that is present in every verb. The verb is at least two syllables long. The four rightmost morphemes in the word, bolded above in Table 1, are the verb stem (X) and the morphemes from the position classes IX (the misnamed 'classifiers'), VIII(subject) and VII(Mode). Together these morphemes are at least two syllables long and comprise the obligatory parts of the verb. Thus, these two syllables contain all the obligatory morphosyntactic specification in these positions. They contain the paradigmatic forms that are the foundation of the verb, the Base Paradigms (g200-201) and the verb theme (g318-356) which is the classifier + stem combination; we will return to these topics in sections 6.3.2 and 6.3.3 respectively.

Table 42 The template of Young and Morgan 1987: g37-38 divided into domains, with the positions in roman numerals (also see Table **6**). The basic obligatory morphemes are on the right edge and are bolded.

Disjunct Domain	Conjunct Domain	Verb Stem
0 Ib Ia Ic Id II III	IV V VIa VIb VIc **VII VIII IX**	X

In (2) is a fully inflected verb form in its minimal size of two syllables. The form listed in the Base Paradigms (g200) in the1st person singular cell of the ø-imperfective paradigm is *yish-* , the classifier + stem combination is - dlá, listed in the stem list (Appendix V) as -DŁÁ (d-dlá) (YM list the stems in capitals, and I observe this convention.)

(2)   yish dlá
           [(y)ish   ] [D   dlá   ]
           [øimp/1s] ['cl' 'drink'   ]
           [VII/VIII] [IX   X (stem)]
           [Aux   ] [Verb   ]
           'I drink it' (YM:g206, column 1)

The 'classifier' prefix, (position IX) has an unusual prosody and surfaces as an onset very rarely. It surfaces as a coda for the penultimate syllable, or it is deleted. The classifier is the locus of the Athabaskan 'd-effect,' and the phonology of the classifier prefix is an area of interest to many linguists. (In example (2) above, it is deleted. This is considered an instance of the 'd-effect'.)

Because all verb forms are built on these two syllables, the Base Paradigms and the classifier-verb stem combination are key to understanding the structure of the verb.

There is no absolute agreement on the number and kind of 'position classes' or on the features that characterize a given position in the Athabaskan literature. There are differences, for instance, in the number and kind of positions in the template between the 1980 and 1987 Young and Morgan. Despite the similarities between the languages, there are also differences between the characterization of the Navajo template by Young and Morgan 1987 and Rice's Slave grammar (1987), and between Rice 1987 and Rice 2000. It is safe to assume, however, that the template in YM (g38-39) is a working model for the general structure across the Athabaskan languages (For discussion of the status of position class as morphological class, and the template as a generative mechanism, see Kari 1990, Hargus 1986, Rice 2000, Axelrod 1992, Faltz 2000, McDonough 1990, 2000a, 2000b).

6.2.2 Epenthetic Elements

There are several instances of epenthetic or inserted segments in the grammar and in the literature in general, and these can be divided into two groups: phonological epenthesis and morphological epenthesis. Phonological epenthesis is the insertion of a consonant or vowel to fill out a phonological constraint. An example is the initial glide in the form in (2) above. The glide only shows up when this morpheme is at the left edge of the word, i.e. when there are no other affixes. The glide *y* is epenthetic in the sense that is appears only when the vowel is in initial position in the word, to fill out the syllable constraint. Thus Young and Morgan 1987 often put it in parenthesis as *(y)i-*. In (3) is an example of a *di-* 'inception' from position VIa with the øimperf/3rd singular (y)i-. The combination surfaces as *di-*.

> (3)   di dzééh
>   [d(i)   (y)i   ] [d   dzééh   ]
>   [inception øimp/3s] ['cl' 'breathe']
>   [VIa   VII/VIII] [IX   X   ]
>   [Aux   ] [Verb   ]
>   *'he takes a breathe' (YM87:d331)*

With morphemes such as the 1st optative, *ó*, the glide is *w (= wó)*, when it is the low vowel it surfaces as a back glide, orthographically written as *gh (=gha)*. The glide is a phonological variant of the vowel. Several prefix vowels are also epenthetic, as in (3) above, although a complete demonstration of this is beyond the scope of this discussion (YM:xi, McDonough 1996). Parentheses around a segment in YM paradigms generally indicate the epenthetic status of a segment.

An example of a morphological epenthesis is captured by the terms 'peg element' or 'pepet vowel'. These terms refer to the use of null or zero morphemes. In the template, there can be null morphemes in all (and only) the positions (VII, VIII and IX), the obligatory morphemes before the stem. These null morphemes represent default specifications: respectively, the ø-imperfective or ø-perfective for the Mode position (VII), the 3rd person for the subject position (VIII) and the default classifier (IX)[2]. In the case that the verb is in the ø-imperfective or ø-perfective, 3rd person singular, with the null classifier, the verb will use a default specification: /i/, the default vowel in Navajo. In a morphological model of this type a word that is in the ø-

imperfective 3rd singular in Navajo will have a *yi-* by stipulation, to fill out
the requirement that a word is two syllables long, as in (4).

(4)   (yi) cha
       [ø   ø   ] [ø   cha   ]
       [Mode subject] [Classifier stem   ]
       [VII   VIII   ] [IX   X   ]
       [Aux   ] [Verb   ]

This *yi-* is called the 'peg element' in the literature, but YM do not use
in it this way. In YM this *(y)i* carries morphosyntactic specification and it is
treated as part of a conjugational paradigm. There are several instances of
this in the paradigms they list and we will consider the *(y)i* as a default
specification. For instance in the form in (5) the specification is ø-
imperfective / 3rd singular.

(5)   yi cha
       [(y)i   ] [ø   cha   ]
       [øimp/3s] ['cl'   stem]
       [VII/VIII] [IX   X   ]
       [Aux   ] [Verb   ]

Throughout the text, the characters that are in parenthesis are either
phonologically epenthetic, or they are conditioned morphophonemic
variants; that is to say, the parentheses represent either phonological or
morphological conditioning.

6.2.3 Verb Themes

Another term that is used is '*verb theme*', which appears to relate to the
make-up of meaning units in the verb. The basic unit in the verb theme is
the classifier + verb stem. In the stem index (Appendix V g:318-356), the
stems are listed in sets with their classifiers, thus the name of the appendix:
'Root / Stem / Theme Index'. A verb theme also may include other
prefixes, although it generally excludes agreement. But any morpheme
from any position can be part of a verb theme meaning unit, including
agreement markers (g72). Example (6) shows a verb theme and its
realization as a full form: *sodi-* is a morpheme that relates to prayer (d689),
while the verb stem is *ZIN* 'think', the classifier + stem is *l-zin*, and the verb
meaning is 'pray'.

Much of the reason for the concept of a 'verb theme' lies in the fact that
is hard to see how these elements combine to give the meaning 'pray',
except by convention. The grammar is rife with example such as this one.
Listing the ways in which the morphemes of the disjunct and conjunct

domain are joined into meaning units is a major work of the dictionary. As we can see in (6), the morphemes of the verb theme are discontinuous; other than the classifier + verb stem, the morphemes are not adjacent to each other if we notate them as the position class template model does. While it is a valuable notion, the verb theme is not a structurally defined or formal entity, but rather simply a list of a string of morphemes. Several models use verb themes as a base for word formation, with problematic results (Kari 1992). We will take up the notion 'verb theme' again when we examine Appendix V in section 6.3.3.

(6)   sodis zin

     sodi   (i)   [1   zin   ]

     'relates to prayer'   øimp/1s   ['cl' 'think want']

     Ib/VIa   VII/VIII   [IX   X   ]

                  D/Aux   [Verb   ]

     'to pray'

6.2.4 The Verb Prefixes

An overview of the position class template (recall Table 6 and Table 42) with a listing of the morphemes assigned to each position is found on pages g37-38. The section of the grammar following this template is called 'The Verb Prefixes' (g39-138). This section is an important reference section in the grammar. It includes remarks on each of the morphemes that are listed in the template with examples of their use. The section is well laid out and fairly easy to follow, though the pages have no headers that indicate what prefix position or morpheme is under discussion. It is easy to lose orientation in the section as discussions of a prefix group may extend for several pages. The Table of Contents is quite helpful as an orientation guide throughout the section.

'The Verb Prefixes' begins with a three-page overview of the structure of the verb that includes a description of the terminology and some of the more general alternations that the consonants and vowels undergo in the paradigms. Morphemes are listed by the position they occur in: the section entitled position VIb, headed "Adverbial–thematic"(g81) lists all the morphemes with the distribution of this position class, with examples of their use.

There is a great deal of homophony among the prefixes of the disjunct and conjunct domain. The homophony rises from the fact that the conjunct morphemes in particular have severely reduced phonemic contrasts; all manner and place features are neutralized and the set of consonantal contrasts among the conjunct prefixes is only slightly larger than that of English inflectional morphemes. The vowels are also quite reduced: *i-* is the default vowel in Navajo, and *Ci-* is the primary syllable shape in all but the

Base Paradigms (see Section 6.3.2). The 'Verb Prefixes' section of YM treats each morpheme separately. For instance, Pos VIb is the position for the various *ni-* morphemes. The template lists seven *ni-* and three *ní-* morphemes, ten total. A discussion of each of these by number begins on page g96. In (7) are three *di* homophones as they are listed in the template for position VIb (g38), and Figure 50 shows the reference entry for *di-*[9] in the section of 'The Verb Prefixes' (g81).

(7)   di-[9] (thematic)   a component of themes involving sanctity, ceremonial
                                      immunity, faith, holiness, respect
         di-[10] (thematic)   relates to color
         di-[11] (thematic)   tilt, slant dangle, be on edge

The entry in Figure 50 is short compared to many of the entries, some of which extend for several pages. I have found it helpful to index the morphemes of the template (g37-38) with the page numbers indicating where they are discussed in the text. Note the numbering of prefixes can be a point of confusion between the grammar and dictionary sections of *The Navajo Language*. The number associated with the prefixes in the template (g37-38) relates only to The Verb Prefix section: this numbering system is not the same as the one used with the prefixes in the dictionary.

```
di-⁹ Ñd-: a thematic prefix that appears in verb themes
that are concerned with holiness, faith, respect, im-
munity from the effects of ceremonies. Dissįįh/dííssįįd,
acquire faith in it (a religion, medical practice);
sodiszin/sodeeszįd, pray.
```

Figure 50 Reference entry for di-[9] (YM:g81)

This section of the grammar also addresses two important topics. First, there are subsections in this section called 'Inventory: Verb Bases', which are part of the entries for several of the position classes. See, for example, pages g86-92. This subsection lists the constructions (called 'Verb Bases') that the various homophones of the morpheme *di-* are involved in. Constraints exist on the mode and aspect that particular verbs may be conjugated in, depending on the morphemes and morpheme combinations present in the verb. The 'Inventory: Verb Base' sections lay out the aspectual paradigms that a given morpheme combination may occur in. The aspectual grammar is a difficult part of the morphology; I will touch on it only briefly, otherwise I refer the reader to the sections in YM on aspect.

Second, 'The Verb Prefixes' section also contains the first discussion of the Modes in the verb (g144-164). These Mode morphemes of Position VII are one of the two morphemes that make up the primary or Base Paradigms (g200-201), (the other is the subject markers of Pos VIII). I have given an example of the partial entry for the si-perfective Mode morpheme from Pos

VII in Figure 47 above. As we can see, this discussion describes the 'deletion' of the *si*-morpheme in the si-perfective Mode. It is important to point out that YM do not use this deletion in their word formation processes, that is to say this entry is not intended to describe a phonological or morphological process. This entry simply is a description of the distribution of this morpheme within its conjugation. The full description of this Mode conjugation is laid out as a paradigm (si-perfective, ø-ł) in the Base Paradigm appendix (g:201), and as we will see, it is this paradigm that is the base of the word formation under YM's own account. While this section on the verbal morphology is an excellent and invaluable guide to the morphemes of the template, it is primarily a reference section, and not a model of word formation.

6.2.5 Aspectual Grammar, Neuter Verbs and Time.

This section is the densest section in the grammar. It runs from pages 164-189, and like the rest of the grammatical sketch is full of examples. The Aspect section is a general discussion of the ways that Navajo builds its aspectual meaning. The aspect morphemes are generally but not exclusively the morphemes of position VIa, VIb and VIc. The section is followed by one on the neuter constructions ("The Neuter Verbs") and an informative section on time in Navajo, ("The dimension of Time in the Navajo Verb" (g202-5)), which sits between the base Paradigms and the Model Paradigms which are important to the formation of the verb word. A full discussion of these sections is beyond the scope of this chapter; I refer the reader to YM.

6.3   THE APPENDIXES

The 1987 grammar has eight distinct appendixes (the 1980 version has 3), listed in Table 43 below. The appendixes appear at the end of the grammar section, between the grammar and dictionary, pages g205-436, and they run half the length of the grammar.

Table 43 Appendixes of YM87

1	Word order	205-205b
2	Appendix I: *The model paradigms*	206-250
3	Appendix II: *The Classificatory verbs*	251-263
4	Appendix III: *Comparative Athapaskan Root inventory*	264-301
5	Appendix IV: *Stem Index*	302-317
6	Appendix V: *Root/ Stem/ Theme Index*	318-356
7	Appendix VI: *Noun Inventory*	357-435
8	Appendix VII: *The Adjectivals*	436-437

The appendixes are the heart of the grammar, providing explicit information in the form of charts and indexes about the morphemes as they occur in Navajo words. For the greater part they are concerned with the semantic properties and phonological shapes of verbal stems in their various aspects (appendixes I, II, III, IV and V). This information is an essential substrate to the dictionary as well as to the grammar. In this section I'll provide a guide for using the two most important appendixes, Appendix I: The Model Paradigms and Appendix V: Root/ Stem/ Theme Index. These are the two paradigms that serve as the base of all word formation. Forms from these two paradigms comprise the final two syllables of the word and the minimal specification necessary to a verb in Navajo.

6.3.1   The Model Paradigms

Appendix I ('Model Paradigms') is useful both for the explicit map of the verb structure it provides and for the examples that are provided. This appendix consists of a list of the verbal paradigms for each of the seven modes listed on pages 200-1 (the 'Base Paradigms') and any possible morpheme (conjunct and disjunct) combination that appears in that mode. Examples of each combination are listed in the bottom section of each page under 'Lexical Examples' and are associated to the paradigms by number. Because of the richness of this information, I'll spend some time discussing this appendix and its accompanying 'Base Paradigms'.

6.3.2   The Base Paradigms

The 'Base and Extended Paradigms' on p200-1 are important in understanding the morpheme structure of a Navajo verb. There are 16 base paradigms that constitute the 16 possible conjugations that a verb form may appear in. Young and Morgan explicitly state: "The 16 Base and Extended Paradigms constitute the foundation upon which all verb bases are conjugated." (g200). A morpheme from a cell in these paradigms combines with the verb stem to form the obligatory part of the verb: the verb stem and the marking for mode and subject. These two morphemes, a 'Base paradigm' morpheme and the verb stem, account for the characteristic bisyllabicity of the Athabaskan verb. In Table 44 are several cells from the Base and Extended Paradigm for the two si-perfective Modes.

The Base Paradigms are a portmanteau of the prefix positions VII and VIII, the Mode and the Subject position classes. Although some of these forms are transparent (such as the 1st Dual), there is enough variation among these forms to require their listing as conjugational paradigms.

The 1st – 3rd singular and dual forms of the two s-perfective Modes are listed in Table 44. The 1st – 3rd person forms are marked 'Base'. The forms marked "3o, 3a, 3i, 3s" are called 'Extended' in Young and Morgan (1987:200). The difference between the base and extended forms are that the Extended forms include morphemes from other positions in the template. The extended base forms in the paradigm in Table 44 include object marking. The forms are the 3rd singular forms that appear with 3rd singular object agreement markers [*j(i)-*, *'(a)-*, *h(o/a)-*], from Pos IV. These 3rd person agreement markers carry semantic marking for the kind of object: general (o), animate (a), inanimate (i), and space/area (s). See the text for examples of these (Young and Morgan 1987:74ff) and discussion of their meaning.

Table 44 Si-perfective paradigm charts (partial) in Appendix I (YM:g201).

II. Perfective			
Base vs. Extended	**Person**	**SI**	
		ø /Ł	**D/L**
BASE	1.	s-é-ø	si-s-
	2.	s-íní-	s-íní
	3.	si-ø	(yi)-s-ø
EXTENDED	3o.	(y)iz- (-s)	---
	3a.	ji-z- (-s)	ji-s-
	3i.	'a-z- (-s)	'a-s-
	3s.	ha-z- (-s)	ha-s-
BASE	1dual	s-ii(d)	s-ii(d)
	2dual	s-oo-	s-oo(h)-

In addition to these forms, Young and Morgan include as an Extended Base Paradigm, forms with the distributive plural, which include the disjunct (non-adjacent) morpheme *da-* , and the Base and Extended Passive forms for each mode. Fully inflected forms using the s-perfective appear in examples (8) through (12). (8) and (9) use the null (ø-) and *ł* - classifiers and the *sé* form of the s-perfective (sperf/1st); (10) and (11) demonstrate the *d*-classifier and the *sis* form of the s-perfective (sperf/d/1st) (the reflexive *'adił* requires the *d*-classifier). The alternations between *s* and *sh* in (9) are a result of regressive consonant harmony.

(8)   sé łtł'is
       [sé   ] [ł   tł'is   ]
       [sperf/1s] ['cl' 'make hard or stiff']
       [VII/VIII] [IX   X   ]
       [Aux   ] [Verb   ]
       'I packed it, made it hard' (YM87:d777)

(9)   shé chíí
        [sé   ] [ø   chíí   ]
        [sperf/1s] ['cl' 'make red'   ]
        [VII/VIII] [IX   X   ]
        [Aux   ] [Verb   ]
        'I reddened it, painted it red' (YM87:d779)

(10)   'adił dah sis tą́
        'adił dah # [sis   ] [d   tą́   ]
        reflex 'on' # [sperf/1s   ] ['cl' 'handle a slender stiff object']
                    # [VII/VIII   ] [IX   X   ]
                    # [Aux   ] [Verb   ]
        'I pinned it on myself' (YM87:d694)

(11)   bił sis zee'
        bił   # [sis   ] [d   zee'   ]
        'to it' # [sperf/1s] ['cl' 'move rapidly']
                # [VII/VIII] [IX   X   ]
                # [Aux   ] [Verb   ]
        'I went as fast as possible' (YM87:d688)

Thus the Base paradigms are a portmanteau of Mode/subject; we will consider a form such as *sé-* to occupy a cell in the s-perfective paradigm, a cell marked for 1st singular. Thus the *sé* is the 1st singular form of the s-perfective (ø/ł) Base Paradigm (=sperf/1st). The (y)ish- is the 1st singular form of the ø-imperfective Base Paradigm (=ø-imp/1st), etc.. These paradigms are conjugational in nature and, as Young and Morgan state, they are the base of word formation. These forms constitute one of the two parts that make up a fully inflected verb and they are the foundation of the Model Paradigms of Appendix I.

6.3.3   The Model Paradigms of the Verb

Appendix V is entitled "The Model Paradigms of the Verb". This appendix and the stem index are the two primary paradigms that constitute a fully inflected word. That is to say, a form from one of these paradigms, in conjunction with a classifier + verb stem will give you a fully inflected Navajo word. The Model Paradigms are in effect instructions on how to put the verb together. The combinations are governed by aspectual and semantic constraints, a topic which is beyond the scope of this chapter. However, this information is available in the grammar, in the appropriate sections (in particular the sections on aspect (g164-189) and the sections entitled 'Inventory: Verb Bases' as discussed above (Section 6.2.5).

In these Model Paradigms each of the sixteen Mode conjugations of the Base Paradigms are listed in separate numbered columns with all the possible disjunct and conjunct combinations. In Column 1, for instance, are listed the Base Paradigm for the ø imperfective, as it is given on page g200. In fact, the Base Paradigm for each Mode is listed in the first column at the beginning of each Mode's listings. For example, the ø-imperfective / Usitative covers columns 1-96 (1987:206-13). The yi-ø imperfective / Usitative starts on column 97 (1987:214) beginning with its Base Paradigm. (Column 97 is the same paradigm that is listed on page 200.) The columns following 97 are lists of the phonological shapes that the various combinations of disjunct and conjunct morphemes respectively take when they are joined with this Mode. That is to say, that the Base Paradigms are the base for the Model Paradigms; they are the form that the prefixes attach to, as shown in (12).

(12)   Prefixes$^{n..\,n+1}$ +Base Paradigms → Model paradigms

The example column in Table 45 gives the shape of the combination of two disjunct prefixes, from positions Ib and Id (*Cé / í + ná*) as they appear for each person / number combination. This column is built on the Base paradigm for the ø-imperfective (1987:g200). The 'C' in the paradigm chart stands for any consonant. The header indicates that the result of the combination of the two listed morphemes (*Cé / í + n*) may be *Céé-*. This form then will combine with the verb stem or the verb theme (the term used to mean the classifier + verb stem combination) to produce a word.

Table 45 A paradigm column entry (YM87:g207) for the forms that combine the ø-imperfective / Usitative Mode with the disjunct morphemes of the shape Cí or Cé plus *ná* by subject marking.

Person / Number	ø-Imperfective/Usitative + Disjunct prefixes 13
	Base paradigm + -Céé = Cé- / Cí Ib + ná- Id
Singular 1.	-Cénásh-
2.	Cééní- / Cénání-
3.	-Céná-
3o.	-Cénéí-
3a.	-Cééjí-
3i.	-Céé'é-
3s.	-Cééhó-

(13)   -Cénásh-
         Ci ná # [ish   ]
                # [øimp/1s]
         Ib Id # [VII/VIII]
                # [Aux   ]

Thus the form in the cell for the 1st singular is listed as -*Cénásh*-; it can be glossed as in (13) as indicated in the header. This form may then be added to a verb unit (classifier + stem). Forms that demonstrate these paradigm morpheme combinations are listed beneath the paradigms at the bottom of the page, under "Lexical Examples." For column 13 above, Young and Morgan list 4 example forms, two related transitive forms with the verb theme ø + *chid,* listed under the stem *CHÍÍD* 'to act with arms or hands' in Appendix V, the 'Root / Stem / Theme Index' (1987:g320); the composite form means 'put arms around his neck'. Two forms with the stem *łóós* ('lead one animate object' (1987:g337)) are combined with verb themes into a form meaning '*ahénáshóós* 'I lead it (animate object) around in a circle'. I give, in (14), an example of one of the pair of the forms, as it appears in Young and Morgan (YM87:g207), with the stem *chid*. The difference between the two forms is the person and number marking of the subject, 1st person (*(i)sh*) versus 3a (3rd animate) (*j(i)*). The second form in the pair is from the 3a cell of the paradigm, an 'Extended Base', as in Table 44. (15) and (16) provide more detail on the morphemes underlying the surface forms in (14).

(14)   bizénáshchid (ø) (vi)   put arms around him   uses 1. -Cénásh-
         bizééjíchid (ø) (vi)   he puts arms around him   uses 3a. -Cééjí-

(15)   bizénásh chid
         bi- zénásh   -chid
         bi- Ci ná # [ish   ] -chid
                    # [øimp/1s]
             Ib Id # [VII/VIII]
         '*put arms around him*'

(16)   bizééjí chid
         bi zééjí   chid
             Ci ná # [ji   ]
                    # [øimp/3a]
             Ib Id # [VII/VIII]
         '*he puts arms around him*'

The glosses in (17) and (18) are derived from the dictionary entry in Young and Morgan (1987:d262). In keeping with the Young and Morgan conventions, the dictionary entry is given in the ø-imperfective, 1st person singular form of the verb, as in *bizénáshchid.*

(17)   bizénásh chid

    bi   zé(é)   ná   # [(i)sh   ] [ø   chid   ]

    'his' 'mouth,throat' 'around' # [øimp/1s] ['cl' 'act with hands or arms']

                                      # [VII/VIII] [IX X   ]

                                      # [Aux] [Verb   ]

    'I put my hands around his neck'

(18)   bizééjí chid

    bi   zé(é)   # [jí   ] [ø   chid   ]

    'his' 'around,mouth,throat' # [øimp/3a] ['cl' 'act with hands or arms']

                                        # [VII/VIII] [IX X   ]

                                      # [Aux] [Verb   ]

    'he put his hands around his neck'

Note that in the 3rd singular animate form, in (18), the *ná* morpheme does not surface: instead the vowel is long, *bi-zéé--*. This alternation is represented in the paradigms. This alternation pattern is not recoverable from the morpheme concatenations in the template. Morpheme concatenations like (*Cé / í + ná = Céé-*) elude clear phonological motivation and are the source of the Athabaskan language family's reputation for morphophonemic complexity. I use the term *polysynthesis* to refer to this type of non-phonological or opaque combination of morphemes. While it is not the case that all morpheme combinations are opaque in the way this one is (in fact the *Céé-* can be separated from the Base Paradigm ø-imperfective quite easily), the paradigms represent sets of clearly related morpheme combinations. From these paradigms it is possible to discover what the surface true morphemes might be, and to deduce consistent patterns that may underlie word formation principles (such as the separation of the disjunct from the conjunct morphemes).

These paradigms are repeated in the dictionary part of the grammar. In the dictionary, Young and Morgan lay out the many paradigms for polysynthetic morpheme combinations that are based on the "Base Paradigms" (1987:200) and the Model Paradigms (1987: 206-50). For the form above, *bizénáshchid,* the individual paradigms for that form, and forms that pattern like it, are listed on page d263 (This number appears at the margin beside the dictionary entry in parenthesis as reference.). These forms appear pretty much as they do in Table 45, with the exception that a particular morpheme, *bizé,* is used instead of the (*Cé / í + ná = Céé-*). We'll take up a discussion of the structure of the dictionary entries in the section 6.4.

6.3.4   The Classificatory Verbs

There are three appendixes that address the verbal morpheme that is the 'content' part of the verb, the verb stem. Navajo stems characteristically carry rich semantic specification that often refers to physical properties of objects such as 'solid roundish', 'flat flexible', 'in an open vessel', 'mushy'. Thus, the physical properties of an object are the content base of a verbal form. This quality, referred to as 'classificatory', is common throughout Athabaskan and other Amerindian languages. It gives them a very distinct semantic profile, and makes translations often difficult. In describing an event for instance, different verbs can be used to describe the same event depending on the point of view you take or the object you are talking about. In Appendix II, *'The Classificatory Verbs'* (g251-263), Young and Morgan lay out the classificatory verbs in charts, and provide a key to how these verb stems are used with objects.

Appendix II is a 13-page chart of objects ("screwdriver", "worm", 'scissors") listed in rows, and the verb stems that are used to talk about them (listed in columns). Given that Navajo has only about 500 stems, this appendix provides an important map of objects and events in the world onto those stems. This section of the grammar also is an important place to begin to learn the aspectual system of Navajo, since the physical properties of an object often preclude or imply certain aspectual relationships that then affect the paradigms the verbs appear in. For instance, to talk about a butterfly, Young and Morgan note that the verb stem used for this will change according to point of view. Butterfly is given a row in the table (g252), and the stem forms are found by reading across the row to locate columns marked by letters, in this case, ABCD. The column indicates that this is a single animate object, and the letters inform us that any of the three stems in this column can be used. The choice of three stems in this column depends on three categories of relationship for that object: handle, drop, or fall. In addition, Young and Morgan note which plural stems can also be used for butterflies. Note that there are no letters for this row in the columns for eating, for instance, as butterflies are not generally eaten.

Another example is the entry 'cactus'. In talking about a cactus, the verb stems one uses will depend on the shape of the cactus, as either flat-leafed (solid, roundish stem), long-stemmed (slender, stiff stem), or domed (solid, round stem), as well as one's relationship to it in an event (handle, drop, fall).

6.3.5   How the Stem Indexes Work

Appendix V (g318-35), like 'The Model Paradigms' appendix, is a basic tool in constructing verb forms. It is an index to the verb themes associated to each verb root. I used the term 'root' here to indicate the abstract form of a stem, since all the stems are marked for aspect. In this index, the roots are entered in their perfective stem forms. They are also capitalized. Thus *CHÍÍD* is the entry form for the verb theme *ø-chid* in (15) and (16) above. In Table 46 are the verb units listed for this entry. I have given the entries as they are in the text but I have included only one example for each theme, though Young and Morgan provide several in many instances. In this entry, there are seven sets of verb themes, and the elements of each set are comprised of a classifier + stem combination and the stem shape for each of the different aspects that the verb theme may appear in (I = imperfective, R = repetitive, P = perfective, F = future, O = optative, Mom. = momentaneous, Con. = continuative.). Note that one of the verb theme stem sets (*lchid (I), (Rep.)) contains a single stem shape in the imperfective. I have bolded the imperfective form in each set.

Note the form *yíníishchiíd*, which is listed as an example in the first stem set in Table 46. This form can be found in the dictionary as an entry (d769). The dictionary entry is given in Figure 51. The final line of the entry tells us that the classifier + verb stem *øchííd* is combined with the prefix group *yíníi-*. This division between the stem and the preceding complex is the primary division in the word[3], and is essential to the way the words are constructed (In fact, this is the single place in the word where consonant cluster may appear).

In this way the inflected word is a combination of the forms from two distinct paradigm types: the prefix paradigms -the Model Paradigms- and the classifier + stem – the 'verb theme' paradigms of the Root / Theme / Stem Index - as in (19).

Table 46 Listing for CHÍÍD in Appendix V, with seven verb themes (YM:g320)

- CHÍÍD: to act with the fingers, hands or arms.
*øchííd (I), *øchi' (R), *øchid (P), *øchił (F), *øchííd (O)   (Mom.) (Yíníishchiíd, to make a grab for it. ...)
*øchid (I), *øchi' (R), *øchid (P), *øchił (F), *øchid (O)   (Rev.) (Bináshchid, to embrace him.)
*(d)chid (I), *(d)chi' (R), *(d)chid (P), *(d)chił (F), *(d)chid (O)   (Rev.) ('Ádináshchid, to put one's arms around oneself.)
* lchid (I),   (Rep.) (Bídíshchid, to tease him, tantalize him,...)
*lchííd (I), *lchi' (R), *lchid (P), *lchił (F), *lchííd (O)   (Mom.) (Bik'idiishchííd, to place one's hand on it,....)
*łchid (I), *łchi' (R), *łchid (P), *łchił (F), *łchid (O)   (Con.) (Naashchid, to gesture with the hands.)

Recall that the base of the Model Paradigms, as YM state (g200), are the forms of the aspect conjugations of the Base Paradigms (recall (12)).

(19)   [Model Paradigm] + [Verb theme] → Verb word

The dictionary lists the 1st person form of the five aspects, the same five we see in the stem index in Table 46, except that the dictionary gives fully inflected word forms. In this way the dictionary and the stem index of Appendix V work together. The dictionary lists the particular word forms that the stem sets of the stem index appear in; that is to say, it combines the stem paradigms and the prefix paradigms.

```
yíníishchiííd (I), neíníishchi' (R), yíníichiid (P), yídínéesh-
     chił (F) yínóoshchiííd (O) (ø), to grab for it, to make a
     grab for it. Dibé yázhí bił dishdeełgo yíníichid ń⁻t'éé'
     tsin bik'ą́ą́h deeshchid, I hit my hand on a stick when I
     grabbed for the lamb. / …
          (*øchiíd: to act with the hands, reach.) (yínii-)
```

Figure 51 The dictionary listing for yíníishchiííd (YM:d769). Note that only one example sentence of the several than YM provides is included.

Let's take another example. The verb stem *-TEEH* appears in several different forms and combines with the classifiers to form verb themes. One of its meanings is 'to move or handle an animate object' (g:342). The first stem set in the listing for *TEEH-* is (*øteeh (I)), and the example form *nishteeh* 'to lie down, recline' is provided. If we turn to the dictionary, we find that there are two homophonous forms for *nishteeh*: the first is *nishteeh* 'I bring it' and the second is *nishteeh* 'I lie down' (d662). In the first form, according to the entry in the dictionary (1978:d662), the verb theme is the transitive *ł-teeh* , and it appears in *ni*-Modal paradigms (ni-imperfective and ni-perfectives). The second *nishteeh,* however, lists the verb theme as *ø-teeh,* and the prefix as *ni-^{5}*, a position VIb morpheme. This *ni-^{5}* morpheme is found as an entry (YM:g658), reproduced as Figure 52.

```
ni-5: Pos.VIb, terminal, connotes that the action of
     the verb ends in a halt or a stoppage.
```

Figure 52 The listing for the prefix *ni-^{5}* (YM:d658).

The two ni- morphemes have different distributional properties. Thus these two homophones of *nishteeh* have different structures: both their verb themes and their prefixes are distinct. This also crucially means that these two forms are associated with different conjugational paradigms, which Young and Morgan note. To see how this works, and to see how the paradigms of 'The Model Paradigms' appendix combine with the stems of the stem index (Appendix V), we will turn to a discussion of the structure of the dictionary in *The Navajo Language.*

6.4   THE DICTIONARY

The dictionary in 1987 *The Navajo Language* makes up the bulk of the book, running over one thousand pages in length. It is primarily a dictionary of fully inflected word forms, though in many respects it is also a theory of the structure of the Navajo lexicon. Besides being word-based, the dictionary has two notable characteristics. It provides extensive paradigms, and the paradigms are an important part of a dictionary entry.

Take for instance the listings for the homophones of *nishteeh*, as discussed in the preceding section. As noted above, the stem is the imperfective – *TEEH* in both forms, but they have different classifiers and are associated with different meanings. The two themes are *ł-teeh* and *ø-teeh*. These two themes do not participate in the same paradigms.

In Table 47 are the two paradigms that YM provide for the two homophones. Note the differences. In the first paradigm, *ł-teeh* appears in the n-imperfective and n-perfective conjugations, from the Base Paradigms, but not si- or yi-. The form nishteeh with the *ł-teeh* base means 'to bring it (an animate object)'. The second form *nishteeh* has the base *ø-teeh* and means 'to lie down' (the animate object is the subject and does the lying down). The form in the second column, the *ni-* morpheme is not part of the conjugation, but it is a prefix added to it. Its distibution is different. The base paradigm in this form is the ø-imperfective, and the words are conjugated differently. Thus there is a difference in a *ni*-Mode and a *ni* morpheme that comes from the prefixes of Pos. VI. The prefix *ni-* does not prevent the verb from appearing in other conjugations, such as the *si*-perfective. The conjugational *ni* does, since it represents the ni-conjugation. I have included the iterative in the tables because the difference is particularly apparent in the iterative (note the difference between the forms for the 1st singular iterative: *náshteeh* and *nánishteeh* respectively). T h e iterative is formed by adding a disjunct morpheme *ná-* to the Base Paradigm in both cases. Table 48 provides a morpheme gloss of the ł-teeh theme.

Table 47 The paradigm entries for the imperfective and iterative of the forms *nishteeh*, with the stem 'to move an animate object' (YM87:d662)

Modes	theme: ł-teeh		theme: ø-teeh	
	imperf	iterative ná	ø imperf	iterative ná
1	nishteeh	náshteeh	nishteeh	nánishteeh
2	níłteeh	nániłteeh	níteeh	nániteeh
3	yíłteeh	nałteeh	niteeh	nániteeh
3o	yíłteeh	néiłteeh	yiniteeh	néiniteeh
3i			'aniteeh	ná'níteeh
3s	hółteeh	náháłteeh		

If we go to the Model Paradigm charts (Appendix I), and look under the n-imperfective, which is listed in column 127 (g216) and labeled as the base paradigm for the ni-imperfective, we will find the forms that are in the first column in Table 48. These Model Paradigm charts also show the Base Paradigm for the n-imperfective, as it appears with disjunct prefixes. The paradigms for a disjunct prefix from position Ib (the position of the iterative) with the n-imperfective are listed in column 129.

Table 48 The 1st, 3rd, 3o, and 3s forms of the base *ł-teeh*, with glosses given.

Modes	imperf			iterative ná				
1	nishteeh			náshteeh				
	nish	ł	teeh	ná #	(ni)sh		ł	teeh
	nimp/1st 'cl' stem			iter. #	nperf/1st 'cl' stem			
3	yíłteeh			nánił teeh				
	(y)í	ł	teeh	ná #	ní		ł	teeh
	nimp/3rd 'cl' stem			iter. #	nperf/3rd 'cl' stem			
3o	yíłteeh			néiłteeh				
	y(i) (y)í	ł	teeh	ná # (y)i	(yi)		ł	teeh
	3o nimp/3rd 'cl' stem			iter. # 3o	nperf/3rd 'cl' stem			
3s	hółteeh			náháłteeh				
	hó (i)	ł	teeh	ná # há	(i)		ł	teeh
	3s nimp/3rd 'cl' stem			iter. # 3s	nperf/3rd 'cl' stem			

Note that the forms of the ø-classifier (ø-teeh) are treated differently. These are the forms associated to the meaning 'to lie down', where the animate object specification refers to the subject of the action. Note especially the 3rd person object forms (3o, 3i, 3s, Young and Morgan, the Extended Paradigms); these include a prefix from Pos V/IV. In these paradigms note the presence of the *ni* between the object agreement marker and the subject marker (Pos. IV) and (VIII); resulting in a different surface form from the paradigm in Table 48.

Table 49 Forms and possible glosses for the 2nd and 3o person forms paradigms .

Modes	ø imperf				iterative ná				
2	níteeh				nániteeh				
	ni	i	ø	teeh	ná #	ni	i	ø	teeh
	term. øimp/2nd 'cl' stem				iter. #	term. øimp/2nd 'cl' stem			
3o	yiniteeh				néiniteeh				
	yi ni	(i)	ø	teeh	ná # (y)i	n(i)	i	ø	teeh
	3o term. øimp/3rd 'cl' stem				iter. # 3o	term. øimp/3rd 'cl' stem			

To see this more clearly, refer to the paradigm charts in the Model Paradigms section (Appendix I, g206). In Table 49, the paradigm charts list the ø-imperfective, not the n-imperfective, as their base. These appear in column 35, where, in addition, we also find forms for *ni-* VIb, the terminative. Column 8 (g210) then gives the paradigm of the iterative forms for the ø imperfective but without this *ni-* prefix. Why? Because inclusion of the *ni-* terminative is quite systematic: the prefix n is subject to phonological and prosodic constraints, as such it is not included among the chart paradigms in the grammar which record primarily difficult or opaque prefix groupings as we have seen (e.g. Table 45 CEE-). However, the paradigm for this form of *nishteeh* is not ignored; it is laid out in the dictionary, on page d656. This is the main point of difference between the dictionary and the Model Paradigms. The model Paradigms in Appendix V handles general conjugational paradigms. The dictionary addresses the structure of the specific words.

At least two essential things can be gleaned from studying the charts and entries in this way. First, generalizations emerge about the possible systematic phonological alternations, as separate from the purely morphophonemic ones. The systematic alternations that are the phonologically or morphologically predictable ones are not generally listed as paradigmatic in the Model Paradigms. The second generalization concerns the aspectual differences between these two forms. The aspectual differences between the forms are expressed in their differing structures: the transitive versus intransitive forms and/or the differences in the distribution of the ni morpheme, between the *ni-* Mode and the terminative (pos, VII versus VI). For the differences between the ni- Mode and the terminative, or between the Mode and the aspectual Pos VI prefixes in general, the reader can turn to the sections in the grammar on the aspectual morphemes (cf. Sussman 2003). In either case, it is an excellent way to begin to understand the aspectual system of Navajo, by reading the dictionary entries and by studying the examples that are given in the entries.

It is important to note that many morpheme concatenations in Navajo words are idiosyncratic; i.e. less than fully compositional. It is also of considerable interest that although Young and Morgan (1980, 1987), Young and Morgan and Midgette (1992) and Young (2000) use a template to lay out the morphemes of the verb, they do not use this template in either the dictionary section or the Appendixes to build their word forms. Instead, paradigms and paradigm charts are used.

6.4.1 Explaining the Paradigms in the Dictionary

Table 50 is a partial paradigm entry from Young and Morgan's dictionary section (1987:d330) for forms that begin with the *di-* morpheme. I have included here only the singular and dual forms, but the full paradigm entry includes a full set of forms. The paradigm in Table 50 is found in the 'd' section of the dictionary, since the words begins with the letter 'd'.

Table 50 Partial paradigm for *di-* (YM87:d330), showing singular and dual.

di- [1,4,5,6,7,8,9,10]

Person	øimp	Iterative	Perfectives			Future	Optative
			si- ø-ł	Si- D-L	Yi- D-L		
1	dish-	ńdísh-	dé-	désh-	díí-	dideesh-	dósh-
2	dí-	ńdí-	díní-	díní-	dííní-	didíí-	dóó-
3	di-	ńdí-	deez-(-s)	dees-	díí-	didoo-	dó-
3o	yidi-	néidi-	yideez		yidíí-	yididoo-	yidó-
3a	jidi-	nízhdí-	jideez	jidees-	jidíí-	dizhdoo-	jidó-
3i	'adi-	ń'dí-	'adeez-	'adees-		di'doo-	'adó-
3s	hodi-	náhodi-	hodeez-	hodees-		hodidoo-	hodó-
1	dii-	ńdii-	dee- (disii-)	dee- (disii-)	dii-	didii-	doo-
2	doh-	ńdóh-	disoo-	disooh-	doo-	didooh-	dohooh-

Across the top of the paradigm the morpheme *di-* is inscribed with the superscripts 1, 4, 5, 6, 7, 8, 9, 10. These superscripts refer to the *di-* morphemes that are associated with these numbers. These numbers are neither position classes nor references to the subscripts in the template (g37-38); they refer to indexes in the dictionary entries. First note that all of these *di* morphemes are homophones in the sense that they have identical shapes and they participate in an identical paradigm. Entries for the individual *di-* morphemes, such as *di-*[1], or *di-*[6,7] are sprinkled unevenly throughout the text, and you can find them by simply searching for them in the vicinity of the paradigm. For instance, the entry for *di-*[1] is found in the first column on page 1987:d331, *di-*[6,7] in the first column of page d333. Take for example the entry for the word *dissááś* 'to dribble along in a line', which is listed on page 1987:d332, and repeated here as Figure 53.

```
dissááś(I),dissááś(I),ńdíssas(R),désas(P),dideessas(F),dóssááś
   (O)(ł), to dribble it along in a line, to strew it
   along (as sand dribbled through one's fingers). Bikáá-
   'adání bikáa'gi 'áshįįh désas ńńt'éé' shimá shich'a-
   hóóshkeed, my mopther balwed me out for dribbling
   salt on the table top./…**ł-zááa = =sáás: to handle or move ---
   small particles. Cf. zas, snow, yidzaas to snow.)
   (di-)
                                                        (330)
```

Figure 53 The dictionary entry for dissááś (YM:d332).

At the bottom of the entry, which is in the lefthand column on the page, the figure (330) appears in parenthesis at the center margin. This number then refers to a paradigm appearing on page 330 (specifically, the one reproduced here as Table 50. This is the manner in which entries are associated to paradigms in the dictionary.

A dictionary entry consists of a listing of the verb forms by mode conjugation, as we have seen. For the entry *disśáás*, the entry starts with the forms of the five Modes, Imperfective (I), Repetitive (R), Perfective (P), Future (F), Optative (O), repeated below as (20) (For the meaning, use, and examples of these Modes, see Appendix II (1987:g144-199)):

(20)   dissááས(I), ńdíssas(R), désas(P), dideessas(F), dósááས(O) (ł)

At the end of the dictionary entry is the classifier – stem combination, the verb unit, here *(ł -záás = sáás)*, and its meaning ('to handle small particles'). The final part of the entry also contains the prefixes that are in the construction, here the prefix *di-*, entered in parenthesis as *(di-)*. The *di-* is part of the meaning of the verb 'to dribble along in a line', as such it is part of the verb theme. In this particular entry, the *di-* is not associated with a superscripted number or a dictionary entry, or, thus, a particular meaning. However the '(330)' at the center margin tells us that we can use the paradigms on page d330 (found in table 7) to build the full set of forms.

For some of the *di-* morphemes, there are separate dictionary entries, as indicated by the superscripts. If there are separate entries for these morphemes or morpheme combinations, they can be found scattered throughout the text around the paradigm. The entry for di-[2] is on p. d331, for instance. It is defined as "Pos. VIa, thematic, relates to the arms or legs." Some entries will have (di-[2]) at the end of their entry, referring to this morpheme, i.e. this meaning, as well a reference to this paradigm, (330). This is the role of the paradigms in the dictionary; they are tokens of the Model Paradigm types.

Some of these paradigms will represent morpheme combinations. An example is the paradigm for *dinii-*[1] (page d329). The dictionary entry for *dinii-*[1] is on the bottom of page d328, repeated in (21):

(21)   dinii-[1]: di-ni-, Pos. VIa-b, prolongative + yi-, Pos VIc, semelfactive.

This entry tells us that this *dinii-*[1] is combined of three morphemes, all identified as aspectual morphemes of position VI. These morphemes comprise the prolongative and the semelfactive (for examples of the meaning and use of those aspectual morphemes see Appendix II.)[4] The paradigm for this morpheme group is on page d329. From this paradigm we can determine that this prefix grouping uses the ø-imperfective. To find verb forms that use this paradigm, search the pages around this paradigm for number (329) at the center margin. There are for instance three entries on page d330, with reference (329) at the bottom of their listing.

To return to the entry for *dissáás*, we are now able to construct words. Let's construct the 3rd singular animate, perfective form of the verb. First we need to locate the perfective of *dissáás , (= désas)* from the entry (in Figure 53) and match it to the paradigm chart reference (d330), in Table 50. From the paradigm, we learn that this is the s-perfective conjugation. (Recall the s-perfective 1st singular form with this classifier is *sé-*, from the s-perfective Base Paradigms (g200).) Thus, from the dictionary entry for the perfective form of the verb (*désas*) and the paradigm chart on page 330, we get can read the 3rd person form *jideesas* with the meaning translated in as 'he dribbled it along in a line'. Note the kind of information that these entries encode. We know that the 1st person singular form of the s-perfective is *sé-* (g201). Since the *di-* is a prefix to this form, then we would expect the surface form for the 1st singular to be *disé-* (recall the discussion in Section 3.5.1). The paradigm tells us that the surface form is instead *dé-*.

The prefix combination *di-* + the s-perfective conjugation results in the loss of the *s-* in the s-perfective conjugational paradigm; this is a characteristic pattern of the s-perfective when it is prefixed. This is the kind work that the paradigms charts do; they explicitly lay out all the probable examples of non-transparent alternations, both morphophonologic and semantic.

6.5   SUMMARY

In conclusion, fully inflected words are constructed by joining forms from the two major paradigm types in Navajo: the Model paradigms, or more specific versions of these forms as they are listed in the dictionary (= dictionary paradigms) and the classifier + verb stem, as shown in (22).

(22)   [dictionary paradigms] + [cl + stem] → Verb word.

The juncture between the prefix, represented in the Model Paradigms and the related paradigms in the dictionary, and the classifier + stem is a major juncture in the word. It represents a boundary between the two primary paradigms that comprise the word, the paradigms of the disjunct-conjunct domains (the Model Paradigms), which have as a foundation the Base Paradigms of g200-201, and the classifier + verb stem unit.

The 1st singular ø-imperfective form of a verb is its dictionary entry. If a verb does not have a 1st sing form, then it is given in the 3rd sing.

From an understanding of these two paradigms and their role in word formation, other aspects of the grammar can be explored. For instance, there are differences in the meanings of the morphemes that are dependent on their distribution, conjunct versus disjunct, or the various positions in the disjunct, such as the differences in meaning of the conjunct *ni-* morpheme depending on whether it is associated to the mode conjugations (n-imperfective) or the prefixes of Pos. VI. Another important topic is the aspectual grammar (g164-199), and the referentiality of the words (g251-263). Aspect is a fundamental and distinctive part of the verb morphology, and it can be quite daunting. Aspect is covered in several sections of the grammar portion of *The Navajo Language* and it is an implicit part of every dictionary entry. Understanding the role of the paradigms in word formation provides a ground-work for an examination of this crucial topic. Understanding how the Model paradigms work also allows us to examine and determine the structure of the separate disjunct and conjunct domains, and it is an excellent foundation for establishing the distribution patterns and the phonotactics of the language from which we might deduce a systematic phonology and prosody.

---

[1] *The Navajo Language* is more than a grammar, since it also contains a Navajo - English and English - Navajo dictionary. However, the Navajo-English dictionary is an integral part of the grammar. I will refer to *The Navajo Language* as a grammar in the text. This is distinct from the separate grammar and dictionary sections of the book, as noted.

[2] In its most productive form, the ø classifier is an intransitive marker, making the default specification intransitive.

[3] This is not a claim about the internal structure of the word, only that this juncture is a major break point.

[4] However, some morpheme combinations that appear in the entries do not have separate dictionary entries, such as the *di-*[3] (1987:d330) and the *dinii-*[2] (1987:d329), though they are listed in the paradigms. Generally, this means that this paradigm is associated to an entry or entries, and is not generalizable in either shape or meaning. What is important here is the fact that the prefixes and prefix combinations are all laid out in paradigms, with examples that allow us to build new forms, in an interrelated set of entries and paradigm charts that are further associated with sections in the grammar that provide more examples and detailed discussion.

Chapter 7

CONCLUSION

7.0   THE NAVAJO SOUND SYSTEM

This monograph on the sound system of Navajo is, of course, not a complete study, which is beyond the work of a single monograph or any single linguist. My goal has been to provide a description of the principle factors in the sound system that can be used as a foundation for further work on Navajo and on other Athabaskan languages.

The Navajo lexicon is primarily verbal and inflectional. There is every reason to accept Young and Morgan's elegant perspective that the verb is built of two distinct kinds of paradigms: the paradigms of the verb stem and its 'classifier', and the Base Paradigms (what I have called the 'Aux stem'). The foundation of the Base Paradigms are the 16 mode conjugations, the forms of which are portmanteaus of mode and subject marking; these portmanteaus vary in the form and manner of conjugational paradigms. The Base Paradigms and the Verb comprise the core verb, the minimal, bisyllabic verb. Beyond the core verb are the prefixes which determine syntactic and aspectual properties of the verb (such as the conjunct *s*-seriative, showing that the action indicated by the verb unit is serial), and of the discourse (such as the disjunct *ch'í* specifying that the verbal event takes place out, along a horizontal surface). The system is simple, built of common elements, and thus, essentially, learnable.

I have adopted this basic framework in the bipartite model of the verb, and the phonetics and phonology have been examined within this model. The verb stem has an important status in the word and this is supported by duration and distribution facts. The break between the Verb stem and the pre-stem complex is a clear one, a point of juncture in the word. It was not uncommon, nor was it a speech error, for speakers, using the careful pronunciation provoked by the recording set-up, to pause between the pre-stem and stem complex, that is, between the two parts of the core verb; this pause never occurred at other places in the verb, for any token of any speaker. The pre-stem complex has its own particular characteristics, at every level of the grammar. The two parts of the verb are distinct, with distinct phonetic, phonological, semantic, and syntactic properties, that result in a complex verbal structure, but word formation is basically a simple process.

Several characteristics of the sounds of Navajo are interesting. Some of these, such as the timing and duration profiles of the stem onsets, are due to the prominence of the stem in the word, but some, such as the production of fricatives and their variation in behavior across place of articulation, inform phonetic and phonological theory. Besides capturing the formal relationship of the parts to the whole, studies of this sort also increase our understanding of the possible range of sounds that occur in human languages, and the level of detail that we need to encode in any grammar.

This study would have been impossible without the work of Young and Morgan. *The Navajo Language* is a model of the lexicon of a polysynthetic language, one of the very few functional models of this language type in existence. The Young and Morgan grammars and dictionaries, in their structure, in the details of the word-based entries and in their extensive and interrelated paradigms, represent a well-articulated and elegant theory of the lexicon of a morphologically complex language. It's a brilliant body of work.

APPENDIX A: NAVAJO WORDLISTS

Compiled by :
Martha Austin-Garrison, Navajo Community College, Shiprock NM
Joyce McDonough, University of Rochester, Rochester, NY

These word lists were constructed to exemplify different aspects of the sound system, such as the phonemic contrasts, tonal contrasts within words, the distinction between sounds as they appear in the stem versus conjunct and disjunct domains, and differences in the sizes of the domains in the word.

Wordlist 1: Phonemic Contrasts

This word list was constructed to investigate the phonemic contrasts in Navajo, as we could identify them. Because of the constraints on the sound system imposed by the morphology, the contrasts of the phonemic inventory are confined to the stem morpheme. Since the language is heavily verbal, and since verbs have a distinct structure with many distributional constraints, the notion minimal pairs, as we are used to thinking of them, are difficult to find. We chose to use prefixed nouns in this list. To get as consistent an environment as possible, the 3rd singular possessive prefix *bi* / [pɪ] 'her/his/one's' was used with nouns. In some cases this produced words that were semantically awkward or anomalous for native speakers ('one's water' for instance). But the word list was checked with speakers before the recording session and we did not use words that speakers were uncomfortable with. I did not use tokens containing speech errors or disfluencies in the analyses. Thus not all words are spoken by all speakers, and some words were dropped altogether.

Some of the spelling conventions in these word lists are different from those used in Young and Morgan. The differences are found mainly in the noun prefix vowels and in the representations of some of the velar fricatives. I have adhered to the transcriptions given to me by Ms. Austin Garrison, though she is not responsible for errors in the lists below. Cross references from the words in these lists to entries in Young and Morgan are noted when they are available. Otherwise, any errors in these wordlists are my responsibility.

Stops - unaspirated

bibííh	'(his) deer'	YM:g3
bidił	'(his) blood'	YM:g3
bigish	'(his) digging stick'	YM:g3
bidziil	'(his) strength'	YM:d359
bijį́	'same day'	YM:d489
bijish	'(his) medicine pouch'	YM:d489
bidloh	'(his) laughter'	YM:g3

Stops -aspirated

bitin	'(his) ice'	YM:g3
bikin	'(his) house'	YM:d494
bitsii'	'(his) hair'	YM:g4
bichííh	'(his) red ochre'	YM:g3
kétłoh	'herbs, spearmint'	YM:d493

Stops - glottalized (ejectives)

bit'iis	'(his) cottonwood tree'	YM:g3
bik'is	'(his) friend, companion'	YM:d895
bits'id	'(his) tendon'	YM:d1040
bich'il	'(his) plant'	YM:g3
bitł'éé'	'the same night'	YM:d726

Nasals

hinishná	'I'm alive, I live'	YM:d445
bimá	'(his) mother'	
nahash'ná	'I move, stir'	YM:d531
yii'mas	'we roll'	YM:d775

Fricatives

sęęs	'wart'	YM:g3
bizęęs	'(his) wart'	
bizid	'(his) liver'	YM:g4
shił	'with me'	YM:g8
bizhí	'(his) voice'	YM:g4
łid	'smoke'	YM:g3
bilid	'(his) smoke'	

Glide/ fricative reflexes

sin	'song'	YM:g3
biyiin	'(his) song'	
his	'pus'	YM:g3
hosh	'thorn, cactus'	YM:g3
bihis	'(his) pus'	
bowozh	'(its) thorns'	
baghaa'	'(its) wool'	YM:d1067
gháá'ask'idii	'camel'	YM:d371

Glides (non derived)

biya'	'(his) louse'	YM:g384
'awéé'	'baby'	YM:g4

Labialized velars

kwii	'here'	YM:d512
hwiih	'into him, satisfaction'	YM:d463

Augmentive

łitso	'yellow'	YM:d518
łitsxo	'orange'	
niłtólí	'crystal clear'	YM:d643
yiyiisxí	' he killed it'	YM:d688
yiishjxíí	'I turned dark from the sun'	YM:d861

Aspirated 't' (also vowel contrasts)

bitin	'(his) ice'	YM:g3
biteeł	'(his) cat tail'	YM:g4
bito'	'(his) juice'	YM:g378
bitoo'	'(his) fluid, water'	YM:g378
tó	'water'	
bita'	'in the middle of'	
bitaa'	'(his)father'	

Aspirated 'k'

bikin	'(his) house'	YM:g370
bikee'	'(his) foot'	
bík'á'anilyeed	'help him'	
bokooh	'(his) canyon'	

Vowels:

bíni'	'(his) mind'	YM:g4
binii'	'(his) face'	YM:g4
bitélii	'(his) donkey'	
biteeł	'(his) cattail'	YM:g4
bita'	'in the middle of'	
bitaa'	'(his) father'	
bito'	'(his) fliud, water'	
bitoo'	'(his) juice'	
bijį́įdóó	'from that same day on'	
bijį́	'same day'	
sęęs	'wart'	
sáanii	'older women'	YM:d684
sání	'old one'	YM:d684
kǫ́ǫ́	'here'	
bikǫ'	'(his) his fire'	YM:d499

Wordlist 2. Tone Contrasts

This is word list of verbs was constructed to elicit as many of the tonal contrasts as possible with a word. It was also used in the study of the distinctions between the three domains (disjunct, conjunct and stem) in the verb.

1. Minimal verbs.

1a. L Verb stem

Item	Tone	Gloss	YM ref
yishcha	LL	he cries (I)	YM:d779
yícha	HL	he cried (P)	

1b. H Verb stem

yisdzį́į́s	LH	I drag it (I)	YM:d775
yídzį́į́s	HH	I dragged it (P)	

2. H disjunct clitic: *ch'í* 'out, horizontally'

2a. σσσ

ch'ínísmáás	HHH	I roll it out (I)	YM:d292
ch'íniikááh	HLH	they go out (3+ in a group) (I)	YM:d293
ch'óoshdeeł	HLL	I toss it out (Opt)	YM:g323
ch'íníshdeeł	HHL	I toss it out (I)	

2b. σσσσ

ch'íninishkaad	HLLL	I herd them out (I)	YM:d290
ch'íniníłkaad	HLHL	you herd them out (2nd) (I)	
ch'íninishchééh	HLLH	I drive out (I)	YM:d290
ch'íniníłchééh	HLHH	you drive out (I)	

3. L disjunct clitic *k'i* 'plant, farm', H and L Verb stem (σσσ)

k'idishłé	LLH	I plant it (I)	YM:d507
k'idíłé	LHH	You (sg) plant it	
bił dzidishkaad	LLL	I slap him (I)	YM:d354
bił dzidíkaad	LHL	you slap him	

4. Pre-stem sequences (5 and 6 syllable words)

hahodinishnííh	LLLLH	I talk endlessly (I)	YM:d396
hanáhodinishnííh	LHLLLH	I talk ENDLESSLY (Rep)	YM:d396

Wordlist 3 Pre-stem Complex

This word list was constructed to examining the properties of the disjunct and conjunct domains; the goal was to build words with larger, rather than minimal, conjunct domains. The size limit on the conjunct domain was three syllables. It was used primarily to investigate the differences between the three domains.

biyah 'aniishłį́į́h	I put it in his mind (to cause to desire)	YM: d121
'aniishháásh	I administer a heat treatment	YM:d121
bik'í#hosíní'áh	you blame him (P)	YM:d205
bik'í#hodiish'aah	I accuse him / I'm going to blame him	YM:d206
bik'í#hozhdii'ą́'	to accuse him (handle a solid round object)	YM:d206
bíbiniissį̜įh	I lean him against it (in a standing position).	YM:d169
bidíníshkaad	I separate or cut them out	YM:d169
bidiniiltsood	become addicted to it	YM:d180
dah didiis'éés	put one's foot, hold one's foot move the legs, step	YM:d315
biih dininisht'aah	get one's head stuck in it	YM:d323
biih dineesht'ą́		
na#'nishtin	I give instructions	YM:d558
niná#'níshtįįh	(Rep)	YM:d559

BIBLIOGRAPHY

Alderete, J. (2001). On Tone and Length in Tahltan (Northern Athabaskan). *Proceedings of the 2000 Athabaskan Language Conference*. S. Hargus and K. Rice (eds.), Amsterdam, John Benjamins.

Anderson, S. (1992). *A-morphous Morphology*. Cambridge, Cambridge University Press.

Aronoff, M. (1994). *Morphology By Itself*. MIT Press.

Axelrod, M. (1993). The Semantics of Time: Aspectual Categorization in Koyukon Athabaskan, U of Nebraska Press.

Axelrod, M. (1999). Lexis, Grammar, and Grammatical Change: The Koyukon Classifier Prefixes. Functionalism and Formalism in Linguistics: Volume II: Case Studies. M. Darnell, E. Moravcsik, F. Newmeyer, M. Noonan and K. Wheatley (eds.), John Benjamins: 39-58.

Beckman, M. E. and J. Edwards (1990). Lengthening and shortenings and the nature of prosodic constituency. *Papers in laboratory phonology I: Between the grammar and physics of speech*. K. A. Beckman (ed.), Cambridge, Cambridge University Press: 152-178.

Browman, C. P. and L. Goldstein (1990). Gestural specification using dymanically-defined articulatory structures. *Journal of Phonetics* 18.3: 299-320.

Carlson, G. (1983). Marking Constituents. *Linguistic Categories: Auxiliaries and Related Puzzles*, F. Heny and B. Richards (eds.), D. Reidel: 69-98.

Catford, J. C. (1977). *Fundamental problems in phonetics*. Bloomington, Indiana University Press.

Cho, T, and P. A Keating (2001). Articulatory and Acoustic Studies on Domain-Initial Strengthening in Korean. *Journal of Phonetics* 29.2: 155-190.

Cho, T., A. Taff, et al. (1997). Some phonetic structures of Aleut. *UCLA Working Papers in Phonetics* 95: 68-90.

Crosswhite, K. (2001). *Vowel Reduction in Optimality Theory*, Garland.

Dart, S. N. (1991). Articulatory and Acoustic Properties of Apical and Laminal Articulations. *UCLA Working Papers in Phonetics* 79: 1-155.

Dart, S. N. (1993). Phonetic properties of O'odham stop and fricative contrasts. *International Journal of American Linguistics* 59: 16-37.

de Jong, K. J. and J. McDonough (1993). Tone in Navajo. *UCLA Working Papers in Phonetics*. Kenneth de Jong and Joyce McDonough (eds.): 165-182.

de Jong, K. J. and S. Obeng (2000). Labio-palatalization in Twi: Contrastive, Quantal, and Organizational Factors Producing and Uncommon Sound. *Language* 76.3: 682-703.

199

Faltz, L. (2000). A Semantic Basis for Navajo Syntactic Typology. *The Athabaskan Languages: Perspectives on a Native American Language Family*. T. Fernald and P. Platero (eds.), Oxford University Press.

Faltz, L. (1998). *The Navajo Verb: A Grammar for Students and Scholars*. Albuquerque, University of New Mexico Press.

Farnetani, E. (1997). Coarticulation and connected speech processes. *Handbook of Phonetics*. W. Hardcastle and J. Laver (eds.), Cambridge, Blackwell: 371-409.

Farnetani, E. and D. Recasens (1993). Anticipatory consonant-to-vowel coarticulation in the production of VCV sequences in Italian. *Language and Speech* 36: 279-302.

Fernald, T. and P. Platero, Eds. (2000). *The Athabaskan Languages: Perspectives on a Native American Language Family*, Oxford University Press.

Fujimura, O. and D. Erickson (1997). Acoustic Phonetics. *The Handbook of Phonetic Sciences*. William J. Hardcastle and John Laver (eds.), Cambridge, Blackwell: 65-116.

Goddard, P. E. (1904). Hupa tracings: typescript. *Ethnological Documents of the Department and Museum of Anthropology*. University of California, Berkeley: 300 leaves.

Goddard, P. E. (1905). *The Morphology of the Hupa Language*. Berkeley, University of California Press.

Goddard, P. E. (1905). Mechanical aids to the study and recording of language. *American Anthropologist* 7.4, October-December.

Goddard, P. E. (1907) *The Phonology of the Hupa Language, Part 1*. Berkeley: University of California.

Goddard, P. E. (1907). *The Phonology of the Hupa Language*. The University Press.

Goddard, P. E. (1912) *Elements of the Kato Language*. Berkeley, University of California Press.

Goddard, P. E. (1928). *Pitch Accent in Hupa*. University of California Press.

Goddard, P. and E. Sapir (1907). Kato linguistic data: holograph. *Ethnological Documents of the Department and Museum of Anthropology*. University of California, Berkeley: 11 sheets.

Goddard, P. and E. Sapir (1907). Kato linguistic data: holograph. *Ethnological Documents of the Department and Museum of Anthropology*, University of California, Berkeley.

Golla, V. (1970). *Hupa Grammar*. Ph.D dissertation. University of California.

Gordon, M. (1996). The Phonetic Structures of Hupa. *University of California Working Papers in Phonetics* 93: 164-87.

Gordon, M., B. Potter, et al. (2001). Phonetic Structures of Western Apache. *International Journal of American Linguistics* 67.4: 415-448.

Gunlogson, C. (2001). "Third-person object prefixes in Babine-Witsuwiten." *International Journal of American Linguistics* 67:4: 365-95.

Halpern, A. (1992) *Topics in the Placement and Morphology of Clitics*. Ph.D dissertation. Stanford University.

Hale, K. (1972). *Navajo Linguistics*, I, II, Manuscript. MIT.

Hale, K., E. Jelinek, M. Willlie (2001). Topic & focus scope positions in Navajo, ms., MIT & University of Arizona.

Hardcastle, W. J. and J. Laver (1997). *The Handbook of Phonetic Sciences*. Blackwell Handbooks in Linguistics, Cambridge, Mass., Blackwell.

Hardy, F. (1969). *Navajo Aspectual Verb Stem Variation*. Ph.D. dissertation. University of New Mexico, Albuquerque

Hargus, S. (1988). *The Lexical Phonology of Sekani*. New York, Garland Publishing Company.

Hargus, S. and S. Tuttle (1997). Augmentation as Affixation in Athabaskan Languages. *Phonology* 14.2: 177-220.

Harris, Z. (1945). Discontinuous Morphemes. *Language* 21:121-127.

Hoijer, H. (1943). Pitch Accent in the Apachean languages. *Language* 19:38-41.

Hoijer, H. (1945). *Navajo Phonology*. Albuquerque, University of New Mexico.

Holton, G. (2001). Fortis and Lenis Fricatives in Tanacross Athapaskan. *International Journal of American Linguistics* 67.4: 396-414.

Howren, R. (1971). A formalization of the Aathabaskan 'D-effect'. *International Journal of American Linguistics* 39: 96-114.

Jelinek, E. (1984). Empty Categories, Case and Configurationality. *Natural Language and Lingusistic Theory* 2.

Jelinek, E. (1989). *Argument Type in Athabaskan: Evidence from Noun Incorporation*. Manuscript, University of Arizona.

Jelinek, E., S.Midgette, K. Rice, L. Saxon (1996). *Athabaskan Language Studies: Essays in Honor of Robert W. Young*. University of New Mexico Press.

Jongman, A., R. Wayland, S. Wong (1998). Acoustic Characteristics of English Fricatives: I. Static Cues. *Working Papers of the Cornell Phonetics Laboratory* 12: 195-205.

Kari, J. (1992). Some concepts in Athna word formation. *Morphology Now*. M. Aronoff (ed.), State University of New York Press, Albany: 84-106.

Kari, J. (1989). Affix positions and zones in the Athabaskan verb complex: Athna and Navajo. *International Journal of American Linguistics* 55.4: 424-54.

Kari, J. (1979). *Athabaskan Verb Theme Categories: Ahtna*. Fairbanks, Alaska Native Language Center.

Kari, J. (1976). *Navajo Verb Prefix Phonology*, Garland.

Kari, J. (1975). The disjunct boundary in the Navajo and Tanaina verb prefix complexes. *International Journal of American Linguistics* 41: 330-346.

Kari, J. (1973). *Navajo Bibliography*. University of Arizona Library, Tucson.

Keating, P. (1990). The Window Model of Coarticulation: Articulatory Evidence. *Papers in Laboratory Phonology I: Between the Grammar and Physics of Speech*. Kingston and Beckman (eds.), Cambridge, Cambridge University Press: 451-70.

Keating, P. and A. Lahiri (1993). Fronted Velars, Palatalized Velars and Palatals. *Phonetica* 50: 73-101.

Krauss, M. (1978). Athabaskan Tone. Manuscript. *Alaskan Native Language Center*.

Krauss, M. (1969). On the classification in the Athabaskan, Eyak and Tlingit verb. *Indiana University Publications in Anthropology and Linguistics* Memoir 24: 49-83.

Krauss, M. (1964). Proto-Athabaskan-Eyak and the Problem of Na-Dene I: Phonology. *International Journal of American Linguistics* 30:118-131

Krauss, M. and J. Leer (1976). Proto-Athbaskan-Eyak *y and the Na-Dene Sonorants. *Alaska Native Language Center*, Fairbanks.

Krauss, M. and J. Leer (1981). Athabaskan, Eyak and Tlingit Sonorants. *Alaskan Native Language Center Papers* #3.

Ladd, D. R. (1996). *Intonational Phonology*, Cambridge Unversity Press.

Ladefoged, P. (1968). *A phonetic study of Western African Languages*. Cambridge, Cambridge University Press.

Ladefoged, P. (1971). *Elements of Acoustic Phonetics*. Chicago, University of Chicago Press.

Ladefoged, P. (1993). *A Course in Phonetics*. 3rd ed. Fort Worth, Harcourt Brace Jovanovich College Publishers.

Ladefoged, P. and I. Maddieson (1996). *The Sounds of the World's Languages*. Blackwell.

LaMontagne, G. and K. Rice (1995). A correspondence account of coalescence. *Papers in Optimality Theory, University of Massachusetts Occasional Papers 18*. L. D. J.Beckman, and S.Urbanczyk (eds.), Amherst, GLSA: 211-223.

Leer, J. (1982). Navajo and Comparative Athabaskan Stem List. *Alaska Native Language Center*. University of Alaska, Fairbanks.

Leer, J.(1982). Navajo and Comparative Athabaskan Stem List. *Alaska Native Language Center*. Unversity of Alaska, Fairbanks.

Leer, J.(1979). Proto-Athabaskan Verb Stem Variation. *Alaska Native Language Center*.

Lehiste, I. (1970). *Suprasegmentals*. Cambidge, MIT Press.

Lindau, M. (1984). Phonetic Differences in Glottalic Consonants. *Journal of Phonetics* 12: 147-55.

Lindblom, B. (1986). Phonetic universals in vowel systems. *Experimental Phonology*. J. Ohala and J. Jaeger (eds.), Orlando, Academic Press: 13-44.

Lindblom, B. and I. Maddieson (1988). Phonetic universals in consonant systems. *Language, Speech and Mind: Studies in Honor of Victoria A. Fromkin*. L. M. Hyman and C. N. Li (eds.), London and New York, Routledge: 62-80.

Lisker, L. and A. S. Abramson (1971). Distinctive features and laryngeal control. *Language* 47: 767-785.

Lisker, L. and A. S. Abramson (1964). A cross language study of voicing in initial stops: Acoustical measurements. *Word* 20: 384-422.

Lockard, E. and K. Lockard (1999). Young and Morgan's *The Navajo Language: A Grammar and Colloquial Dictionary* on CD ROM, Salina Bookshelf, Inc., Flagstaff.

Maddieson, I. (1984). *Patterns of Sounds*. Cambridge, Cambridge University Press.

Maddieson, I. (1980). UPSID: UCLA phonological segment inventory database. *UCLA Working Papers in Phonetics* 50: 4-56.

Maddieson, I. (1980). Vocoid approximants in the world's languages. *UCLA Working Papers in Phonetics* 50: 113-120.

Maddieson, I. and K. Emmory (1984). Is there a valid distinction between voiceless lateral approximants and fricatives? *Journal of Phonetics* 41:181-90.

Manual, S. Y. (1999). Cross-language studies: relating language-particular coarticulation patterns to other language-particular facts. *Coarticulation: Theory, Data and Techniques*, William Hardcastle and Nigel Hewlett (eds.), Cambridge University Press: 179-98.

Manuel, S. Y. (1990). The role of contrast in limiting vowel-to-vowel coarticulation in different languages. *Journal of the Acoustical Society of America* 88:1286-1298.

McDonough, J. (2000a). Athabaskan redux: against the position class as a morphological category. *Morphological Analysis in Comparison*. Dressler, Pfeiffer, Pochtrager and Rennison (eds.), Benjamins.

McDonough, J. (2000b). On the bipartite model of the Athabaskan verb. *The Athabaskan Languages: Perspectives on a Native American Language Family.* T. B. Fernald and P. R. Platero (eds.), Oxford University Press: 139-166.

McDonough, J. (1999). Tone in Navajo. *Anthropological Linguistics* 41.4: 503-539.

McDonough, J. (1996). Epenthesis in Navajo. *Athabaskan Language Studies: Essays in Honor of Robert W. Young.* Jelinek, Saxon and Rice (eds.), Albuquerque, University of New Mexico Press: 235-257.

McDonough, J. (1990). *Topics in the Morphology and Phonology of Navajo Verbs.* University of Massachusetts at Amherst.

McDonough, J. and M. Austin-Garrison (1995). Vowel enhancement and dispersion in the Navajo vowel space. *University of California Working Papers in Phonetics.* Ian Maddieson (ed.), 87:105-113.

McDonough, J. and P. Ladefoged (1996). The specification of stop contrasts in Navajo. *Dam Phonology: HIL Phonology Papers II*, Marie Nespor and Irene Vogel (eds.), Holland Institute of Linguistics Publications: 123-142.

McDonough, J., P. Ladefoged, and H. George (1993). Navajo vowels and universal phonetic tendencies. *University of California Working Papers in Phonetics*, deJong and McDonough (eds.), 84:143-150.

Michelson, K. (1988). *A Comparative Study of Lake-Iroquoian Accent.* Boston: Kluwer Academic Publishers.

Morice, A. G. (1932) *The Carrier Language.* Winnepeg.

Ohman, S. E. G. (1966). Coarticulation in VCV utterances: Spectrographic measurements. *Journal of the Acoustical Society of America* 39:151-68.

Pike, E. (1986). Tone Contrasts in Central Carrier. *International Journal of American Linguistics* 52.4: 411-418.

Randoja, T. K. (1989). *The Phonology and Morphology of Halfway River Beaver*, Ph.D. dissertation. University of Ottawa.

Recasens, D. (1990). The articulatory characteristics of palatal consonants. *Journal of Phonetics* 18.2: 267-280.

Rice, K. (2000). *The Athabaskan Verb.* Cambridge.

Rice, K. (1986). *Slave*, Mouton de Grutyer.

Rice, K. (1978). *Hare Dictionary.* Ottawa, Northern Social Research Division, Department of Indian and Northern Affairs.

Reichard, G. (1952). *Navajo Grammar.* New York, J. J. Augustin.

Sapir, E. (1938). Glottalized continuants in Navaho, Nootka and Kwakiutl. *Language* XIV: 248-274.

Sapir, E. (1925). Pitch accent in Sarcee. *Journal de la Société des Américanistes de Paris*, 17:185-205.

Sapir, E. and H. Hoijer (1967). *The Phonology and Morphology of the Navajo Language.* University of California, Berkeley.

Shadle, C. (1991). The effect of geometry on source mechanisms of fricative consonants. *Journal of Phonetics* 19.3/4: 409-424.

Shadle, C. (1985). The acoustics of fricative consonants. *Research Laboratory of Electronics*, MIT.Simpson, J. and M. Withgott (1986). Pronominal clitic clusters and templates.

Syntax and Semantics 19: The Syntax of Pronominal Clitics. H. Borer (ed.), Academic Press.

Smith, C. (2000). The Semantics of the Navajo Verb. *The Athabaskan Languages: Perspectives on a Native American Language Family.* T. Fernald. and P. Plater, (eds.), Oxford University Press.: 200-227.

Speas, M. (1984). Navajo prefixes and word structure typology. *MIT Working Papers in Linguistics* R. Sproat (ed.), Massachusetts Institute of Technology: 134-145.

Sproat, R. and O. Fujimora (1993). Allophonic variation in English /l/ and its implications for phonetic implementation. *Journal of Phonetics* 21: 291-311.

Stanley, Richard (1969). *The Phonology of the Navajo Verb.* Ph.D. dissertation. Massachusetts Institute of Technology.

Stevens, K. N. (1998). *Acoustic phonetics.* Cambridge, Mass., MIT Press.

Stevens, K., S. Blumstein, et al. (1992). Acoustic and perceptual characteristics of voicing in fricatives and fricative clusters. *The Journal of the Acoustical Society of America* 91.5: 2979-3000.

Story, G. L. (1989). A report on Carrier pitch phenomena: with special reference to the verb prefix tonomechanics. *Athabaskan Linguistics: Current Perspectives on a Language Family,* E-D Cook and K. Rice (eds.), Hague, Mouton: 99-144.

Story, G. L. (1984). *Babine & Carrier Phonology.* Dallas, Tex., Summer Institute of Linguistics.

Stump, G. (1992). "Position classes and morphological theory. *Yearbook of Morphology 1992:* 129-180.

Sussman, R. (2003) interpretation and semantic domain: Evidence from Navajo, talk given at the LSA, Atlanta.

Sussman, R. and J. McDonough (2003). Aspect as interaction: *ni* across the regions of the Navajo verb. *University of Rochester Working Papers in the Language Sciences, 3 (1).*

Thompson, C. (1993). The areal prefix 'hu-' in Koyokon Athabaskan. *International Journal of American Linguistics* 59:3: 315-333.

Tuttle, S. (1991). Metrical Structures in Salcha Athabaskan. *Papers from the American Indian Languages Conference,* J. Redden (ed.), Santa Cruz Department of Linguistics, Southern Illinois University Press.

Tuttle, S. (1994). *The peg prefix, the foot and word minimum: evidence from Salcha,* M.S. thesis. University of Washington, Seattle.

Tuttle, S. (1998). *Metrical and Tonal Structures in Tanana Athabaskan.* Ph.D. dissertation. University of Washington.

Willie, M. (1996). On the expression of Modality in Navajo. *Athabaskan Language Studies: Essays in Honor of Robert W. Young.* Jelinek, Saxon and Rice (eds.), Albuquerque, University of New Mexico Press: 331-347

Willie, M. and E. Jelinek (2000). Navajo as a Discourse Configurational Language. *The Athabaskan Languages: Perspectives on a Native American Language Family.* P. Platero and T. Fernald (eds.), Oxford University Press: 252-287.

Wright, R., S. Hargus and K. Davis (2002). On the categorization of ejectives: data from Witsuwit'en. *Journal of the International Phonetic Association* 32.1: 43-78.

Young, R. (2000). *The Navajo verb system : an overview*. Albuquerque, NM, University of New Mexico Press.

Young, R. and W. Morgan (1994). *Colloquial Navaho: a dictionary*. New York, Hippocrene Books.

Young, R., and W. Morgan. (1992). *An Analytic Lexicon of Navajo*. Albuquerque, University of New Mexico Press.

Young, R. and W. Morgan (1987). *The Navajo Languag*. Albuquerque, University of New Mexico Press.

Young, R. and W. Morgan (1980). *The Navajo Language*. Albuquerque, University of New Mexico.

Young, R., W. Morgan, et al. (1976). *The Navaho language : the elements of Navaho grammar with a dictionary in two parts containing basic vocabularies of Navaho and English*. Salt Lake City, Desert Book Co.

Young, R., W. Morgan, et al. (1964). *The Navaho language: the elements of Navaho grammar with a dictionary in two parts containing basic vocabularies of Navaho and English*. Salt Lake City, Utah, Desert Book Co.

Young, R. and W. Morgan (1951). *A vocabulary of colloquial Navaho*. Washington, U.S. Indian Service.

Young, R. and W. Morgan (1951). *Navajo Dictionary*. Washington.

Young, R., W. Morgan, et al. (1946). *The ABC of Navaho*. Phoenix, Phoenix Indian School Printing Dept.

Young, R. and W. Morgan (1943). *The Navaho Language*. Salt Lake City, Education Division, United States Indian Service.

Bibliography

INDEX OF SUBJECTS

Studies in Natural Language and Linguistic Theory

20. H. Lasnik: *Essays on Restrictiveness and Learnability.* 1990
ISBN 0-7923-0628-7; Pb 0-7923-0629-5
21. M.J. Speas: *Phrase Structure in Natural Language.* 1990
ISBN 0-7923-0755-0; Pb 0-7923-0866-2
22. H. Haider and K. Netter (eds.): *Representation and Derivation in the Theory of Grammar.* 1991 ISBN 0-7923-1150-7
23. J. Simpson: *Warlpiri Morpho-Syntax.* A Lexicalist Approach. 1991
ISBN 0-7923-1292-9
24. C. Georgopoulos: *Syntactic Variables.* Resumptive Pronouns and A' Binding in Palauan. 1991 ISBN 0-7923-1293-7
25. K. Leffel and D. Bouchard (eds.): *Views on Phrase Structure.* 1991
ISBN 0-7923-1295-3
26. C. Tellier: *Licensing Theory and French Parasitic Gaps.* 1991
ISBN 0-7923-1311-9; Pb 0-7923-1323-2
27. S.-Y. Kuroda: *Japanese Syntax and Semantics.* Collected Papers. 1992
ISBN 0-7923-1390-9; Pb 0-7923-1391-7
28. I. Roberts: *Verbs and Diachronic Syntax.* A Comparative History of English and French. 1992 ISBN 0-7923-1705-X
29. A. Fassi Fehri: *Issues in the Structure of Arabic Clauses and Words.* 1993
ISBN 0-7923-2082-4
30. M. Bittner: *Case, Scope, and Binding.* 1994 ISBN 0-7923-2649-0
31. H. Haider, S. Olsen and S. Vikner (eds.): *Studies in Comparative Germanic Syntax.* 1995 ISBN 0-7923-3280-6
32. N. Duffield: *Particles and Projections in Irish Syntax.* 1995
ISBN 0-7923-3550-3; Pb 0-7923-3674-7
33. J. Rooryck and L. Zaring (eds.): *Phrase Structure and the Lexicon.* 1996
ISBN 0-7923-3745-X
34. J. Bayer: *Directionality and Logical Form.* On the Scope of Focusing Particles and Wh-in-situ. 1996 ISBN 0-7923-3752-2
35. R. Freidin (ed.): *Current Issues in Comparative Grammar.* 1996
ISBN 0-7923-3778-6; Pb 0-7923-3779-4
36. C.-T.J. Huang and Y.-H.A. Li (eds.): *New Horizons in Chinese Linguistics.* 1996 ISBN 0-7923-3867-7; Pb 0-7923-3868-5
37. A. Watanabe: *Case Absorption and WH-Agreement.* 1996
ISBN 0-7923-4203-8
38. H. Thráinsson, S.D. Epstein and S. Peter (eds.): *Studies in Comparative Germanic Syntax.* Volume II. 1996 ISBN 0-7923-4215-1
39. C.J.W. Zwart: *Morphosyntax of Verb Movement.* A Minimalist Approach to the Syntax of Dutch. 1997 ISBN 0-7923-4263-1; Pb 0-7923-4264-X
40. T. Siloni: *Noun Phrases and Nominalizations.* The Syntax of DPs. 1997
ISBN 0-7923-4608-4
41. B.S. Vance: *Syntactic Change in Medieval French.* 1997 ISBN 0-7923-4669-6
42. G. Müller: *Incomplete Category Fronting.* A Derivational Approach to Remnant Movement in German. 1998 ISBN 0-7923-4837-0

Studies in Natural Language and Linguistic Theory

Kluwer Academic Publishers – Dordrecht / Boston / London